Pain

An Exploration

NORMAN AUTTON

Foreword by Dame Cicely Saunders

Darton, Longman and Todd
London

First published in 1986 by
Darton, Longman and Todd Ltd
89 Lillie Road, London SW6 1UD

© 1986 Norman Autton

ISBN 0 232 51657 X

British Library Cataloguing in Publication Data

Autton, Norman
   Pain : an exploration
   1. Pain
   I. Title
   616′.0472   RB127

   ISBN 0–232–51657–X

Phototypeset by Input Typesetting Ltd
London SW19 8DR

Printed and bound in Great Britain by
Anchor Brendon Ltd
Tiptree, Essex

Dedicated
to

All those, who are any ways afflicted, or distressed, in mind, body, or estate: that it may please thee to comfort and relieve them, according to their several necessities, giving them patience under their sufferings, and a happy issue out of all their afflictions.

Collect or Prayer for all Conditions of Men
Book of Common Prayer (1662)

Contents

Foreword

Writing thirty years ago on the nature and significance of chronic pain, Aring (1956) drew attention to Sophocles' drama, *Philoctetes*, as an illustration of a profound understanding of pain in a culture of over two thousand years ago.

Philoctetes, one of the captains in the Greek forces, suffered a wound on the way to Troy. Abandoned by the Greeks on a lonely isle he is tortured for ten years by the festering wound. He ekes out a bare existence by reason of his possession of the infallible bow of Apolla. Aring quotes, annotated for medical consumption, an analysis of the ensuing drama by the literary critic Edmund Wilson (1941). The Greeks send the young Neoptolemus to seize the bow by cunning, but instead, as a just and guileless young man (the understanding physician), he effects a cure by recognising the wrong (corrects the diagnosis). He is human enough to treat Philoctetes not as a monster (a neurotic nuisance) but simply as another human being whose suffering elicits his sympathy and whose courage and pride he admires (insight into the good in man and alliance with it). When this human relationship has been realised and Neoptolemus becomes aware of his common humanity with the sick man, the stubbornness of Philoctetes is dissolved (his character is altered by the relationship), he is cured – and the Greek campaign is saved as well.

Not all patients with persistent pain are thus fully cured but few fail to be helped by a relationship such as that described by Sophocles. The demands made on those close to pain are well illustrated by some of the comments made to the author by the nurses who responded to a survey reported in Chapter 5. Members of staff concerned with such people, especially nurses, the hands-on carers, have their own needs as they have to come to terms with the impact of someone else's pain. Even the comparatively short-term anxieties of acute pain, the more common hospital experience, with its foreseeable end and built in meaning ('Of course I've got a pain, I've had an operation') can be taxing for all parties. But what of the complexities of chronic pain, with no end in sight nor reassuring meaning? Here patient, family and staff all face problems perceptively described by the author from his many years of experience of such situations. One does not travel by the easy road of indifference to the uplands of toleration (Churchill on Charles II, 1956) but by a careful search for understanding.

This book is an admirable description of such a search and by adding his unusually wide reading to his years as a hospital chaplain, Canon Autton has gathered a wealth of information that will be of value to readers of a variety of professions, and perhaps, too, to people involved with pain in a more personal way. Some will want to turn first to the later chapters but the details of diagnosis and treatment reviewed earlier bring a valuable overview of the present state of this fascinating and changing field.

Man cannot help but search for meaning. Here is a guide to understanding that will go far in sustaining a relationship that is not drained by imprudent over-involvement but instead helps to create a climate in which a patient is sure enough of his worth to make his own search.

Cicely Saunders

April 1986

Aring, C. D.	'The nature and significance of chronic pain, *Med. Clin. N. Amer.*, 42 (1956), p. 1467.
Churchill, W. S.	*A History of the English Speaking Peoples*, vol. II, *The New World* (London 1956), p. 269.
Wilson, E.	*The Wound and the Bow*. Houghton Mifflin (Cambridge, Mass. 1941), p. 295.

Preface

At a recent conference on Pain a radio commentator asked why discussion of such a subject was thought to be necessary. A consultant anaesthetist had a ready answer: 'Because there happens to be a lot of it about!' he replied. Pain is a matter of intense personal interest and concern to almost every one of us. Each year more than 23 million people visit their family doctors, a large percentage of whom present pain symptoms. Advertisements abound both on television and in the press promoting products which offer 'instant relief' from a multiplicity of various aches and pains.

Pain is so familiar an experience that we are inclined to take it for granted, yet it is a subject which has taxed the intellect of theologians and medical practitioners over the years. In an endeavour to understand pain it has been presented as a 'problem' (C. S. Lewis, 1940), a 'puzzle' (R. Melzack, 1973), and a 'challenge' (R. Melzack and P. D. Wall, 1982).

This volume is not intended to be either a theological or a medical dissertation on the subject, but rather an 'exploration' by a non-medical writer who happens to serve as a hospital chaplain within the confines of a large modern Medical Centre, and whose ministry inevitably involves him in the care of a large number of patients who are in pain. No longer can the subject of pain be regarded as solely the preserve of the medical world, for there are many factors involved which lie beyond the limits of the disease process. Pain affects the whole of man.

In the following chapters attempts are made to outline the nature, variety and relief of pain, children and pain, the various attitudes of professional carers and patients, and finally some aspects of ministry. It is hoped that the book will be of interest not only to hospital chaplains and parochial priests and ministers in their pastoral care of sick people, but also to medical, nursing, and social-work students, and all who in their respective roles have to deal with patients in pain.

My thanks have to be extended to a large number of friends in the spheres of both church and medicine, who are too numerous to mention personally. I trust they will be charitable and all feel included in a general vote of most sincere thanks. I must however acknowledge those without whose wisdom, counsel and advice the book would not have been written at all, and express to them my gratitude and appreciation. They include Dr Robert Twycross, Consultant Physician at the Churchill Hospital, Oxford; Dr Keith Murrin, Consultant Anaesthetist, University of Wales Medical College, Cardiff; and Margo McCaffery, Consultant in the Nursing Care of People with Pain, Santa Monica, California, who read the original draft of Chapters 1 to 4, and not only guided me through many of the physiological and psychological intricacies of pain experience, but also made a number of useful and constructive comments.

The librarians of both the University of Wales Medical College Library, and the School of Nursing Library at the Combined Training Institute were most generous in their assistance in the procuring of books, journals and papers dealing with aspects of pain.

I wish to express my most sincere appreciation to Dame Cicely Saunders, DBE, FRCP, Chairman of St Christopher's Hospice, Sydenham, London, for her most generous foreword. Along with countless others I have learned so much about the problem of pain from her teaching and writings.

The Director of Nurse Education at the School of Nursing, and the staff of the Department of Nursing Studies were all extremely co-operative and supportive, and generously arranged for a number of their nursing students to participate in a study of attitudes to pain experiences (Chapter 5). The children in the School of the Department of Child Health very readily responded to questions dealing with their feelings towards pain, and often brought out most illuminating expressions (Chapters 4 and 5).

Finally I must offer grateful thanks to my secretary, Mrs

Anne Taylor, who in labouring over various drafts of the
manuscript must have experienced personally much mental
if not physical pain, yet bore it all cheerfully and without
complaint!

Cardiff, 21 December 1985   Norman Autton
(St Thomas, Apostle)

Lewis, C. S.   *The Problem of Pain*. Fontana, London 1940.
Melzack, R.   *The Puzzle of Pain*. Penguin, London 1973.
Melzack, R., and   *The Challenge of Pain*. Penguin, London 1982.
  Wall, P. D.

Nature of Pain

It would be a great thing to understand pain in all its meanings.

Peter Mere Latham (1789–1875)

I thought I knew what pain was until I was asked to say what the word 'pain' means.

J. J. Degenaar (1979)

Pain is a great paradox. It is replete with anomalies and contradictions. It can be creative and destructive; it can ennoble and embitter; it can protect and destroy. Pain can be a warning sign that something is wrong and yet can diminish the will to live. It can be associated with survival and also with disease and death. Both saint and sinner are prey to it. It is an effect of evil but can also be a means of good.

Pain is a private personal experience common to all individuals yet unique to each. It means significantly different things to different people, in terms of quality as well as quantity, and is extremely difficult to define on account of its complex interactions. In his classic treatise on pain Sir Thomas Lewis (1942) describes the dilemma: 'Reflection tells me that I am so far from being able satisfactorily to define pain, of which I here write, that the attempt could serve no useful purpose. Pain, like similar subjective things, is known to us by experience and described by illustration.' As observers we can play no part in it for no one can fully share the pain of another person; only the individual feels his own pain. Others can only infer or imagine what the experience is like. For information about it we are wholly dependent upon the report of the sufferer himself but no two people will describe similar painful experiences in precisely the same terms. The patient is the authority on his own pain for only he knows what it means to him personally; yet the average person would readily agree with Virginia Woolf (1948): 'English . . . has no words for the shiver and headache . . . the merest schoolgirl, when she falls in love, has Shakespeare and Keats to speak for her; but let a sufferer try to describe a pain in his head to a doctor and language at once runs dry.'

Pain is a great puzzle. It is one of the most complex of all human experiences. The search for an adequate definition has been likened to the story of a group of blind men attempting to describe an elephant; each will understand the shape and size of the elephant as that part of the animal with which he comes into contact. Such diverse disciplines as philosophy, medicine, psychiatry and social anthropology will each have its distinct theories and approaches to the study of the complex problem of pain. The philosopher will be concerned with the sensations: feeling, suffering and meaning; the anaesthetist and surgeon with the physical manifestations; the psychologist with the emotional qualities; the psychiatrist with the mental reactions to stress; and the theologian with aspects of guilt or retribution. In spite of pain being a universal human experience it is well-nigh impossible to describe in words. 'It seems that too much remains to be learned about pain mechanisms before we can define pain with precision' (Melzack and Wall, 1982). One of the major problems is that of semantics. The word 'pain' itself has a variety of connotations, from the agony of a post-herpetic neuralgia (shingles) to a 'painful divorce'; or even to an acquaintance who is dismissed as 'a pain in the neck'.

We can only think of pain experiences in terms which evoke pain. Thus we may say that our pain is 'sharp', thinking of a severe blow or cut; or 'nagging', 'burning' or like a 'pinprick' (see p. 27). One patient related: 'The terrible pain in my left leg was unbelievable – the worst I'd ever experienced – it seemed as if my leg was peppered all over with red-hot pokers shooting in and out.' In their study of words used to describe pain experience Melzack and Torgerson (1971) found 'that the word "pain" refers to an endless variety of qualities that are categorised under a single linguistic label, not to a specific single sensation that varies only in intensity. Each pain has unique qualities. The pain of a toothache is obviously different from that of a pin-prick . . .'. The very fact that there are a multiplicity of words and phrases to describe it lends support to the concept of 'pain' as an overall term which really represents a myriad of different experiences and refutes the traditional idea that pain is a single modality which has one or two specific qualities.

Throughout the centuries the problem of pain has vexed the minds of physicians, philosophers and theologians, and although man has been slow to examine and define it, the desire to investigate pain sense and to evaluate its role in human life is ancient. Aristotle (384–322 BC) excluded pain from his classification of the five senses (vision, hearing, smell, taste and touch) for he considered it to be 'a quale of the soul', a state of feeling and the epitome of unpleasantness. He believed that the heart was the *sensorium commune* and that pain was conveyed by the blood to the heart. Like Plato before him, who suggested that pain was the result of the violent actions of earth, air, fire and water, the four elements of the soul, he placed pain with pleasure among the passions of the soul. 'We measure our actions', stated Aristotle, 'by the role of pleasure and pain.' He believed that pain experience was a negative passion, conquered by reason, and with its natural opposite, pleasure, was the basic moral drive guiding man's actions, 'for moral excellence is concerned with pleasures and pain'. (Compare the condemnation of Eve in Genesis 3:16, 'I will greatly multiply thy sorrow and thy conception; in sorrow thou shalt bring forth children'.) Such was a commonly held view of the problem of pain for some two thousand years until studies of sensory perception in the mid-nineteenth century were placed in juxtaposition to the older emotion theory.

In the early seventeenth century Descartes (1596–1650) accepted the theory that the brain was the seat of both sensation and pain; the conduction of pain was mediated via delicate threads in the nerves which connect the tissue to the brain. Further pain theories were elaborated throughout the seventeenth, eighteenth and nineteenth centuries. Two major theories emerged, in addition to Aristotle's theory which described pain as an 'affective quality'; the 'specificity theory' claimed that pain has its own sensory apparatus independent of touch and the other senses, and the 'intensive theory' propounded that every sensory stimulation of pain is capable of producing pain if it is of sufficient intensity. After decades of discussion and debate over these three theories it was the 'specificity theory' which by the 1950s eventually won general acceptance in the medical and scientific community.

Theology has struggled with the problem of pain from the prophet Job, Song of Solomon, Psalms and Deutero-Isaiah, on to the theme of redemptive suffering in the New Testament, where the vicarious aspect of the suffering servant finds its fulfilment in Christ's passion, death and the final note of victory. The theological problem in its simplest form was stated by C. S. Lewis (1940), who saw the religious significance of pain as the call of God for man:

> When our ancestors referred to pains and sorrows as God's 'vengeance' upon sin they were not necessarily attributing evil passions to God; they may have been recognising the good element in the idea of retribution. Until the evil man finds evil unmistakably present in his existence in the form of pain he is enclosed in illusion. Once pain has roused him he knows that he is in some way or other 'up against' the real universe; he either rebels with the possibility of a clearer issue and deeper repentance at some later stage, or else makes some attempt at an adjustment, which, if pursued, will lead him to religion . . . no doubt pain as God's megaphone is a terrible instrument; it may lead to final and unrepented rebellion but it gives the only opportunity the bad man can have for amendment.

Pain plays a central role in religious thought. It reminds us of the frailty of all that is human. The Christian concept of pain must always be seen as a paradox. On the one hand Christ healed others in pain and proclaimed the miracles as signs of his work of redemption. On the other he allowed himself to be crucified unjustly and to endure the most agonising of pain.

Pain is borne best not with a stoic resignation or submission but as a challenge – an active taking up in defiance. It is not to seek some blissful nirvana but rather to acknowledge its reality. There is to be an active willing conscious acceptance

4

of our share in the pain of the world. In this way pain can be seen as having a positive purpose and value of its own; and it can be creatively handled so that out of it may come a genuine enrichment of life. It is not pain per se which is redemptive but the attitude towards it. The Christian faith neither explains nor justifies pain but rather suggests that there is something to be done about it which men may find it worthwhile to do.

What is not compatible with the Christian ethic are the two extreme concepts: either of avoiding pain at all costs as the greatest of evils, or of glorifying suffering and idealising pain as something good in itself. The cross is the great symbol of the meaning of pain and it is there that many find comfort and hope in loneliness and despair. (It is interesting to note that the description of pain as 'excruciating' is derived from the practice of crucifixion itself.) To attempt to avoid suffering at all costs leads only to an increase of pain, for the more we try to avoid it the lower our threshold of resistance becomes. It is in facing and accepting pain that it is overcome. The concept that some pain is unavoidable should not degenerate into a mere excuse for tolerating avoidable pain. Although pain may stimulate reflection and strengthen character the Christian attitude is compatible with the desire to avoid pain.

The distinction between pain and suffering is not always clear, for there are many psychological factors involved. Hick (1968) observes that 'the extent to which a given quantity of the pain sensation causes us to suffer, and comes to determine the quality of our consciousness, varies enormously both from person to person and from time to time for the same person'. Pain undoubtedly causes suffering but not all suffering is due to pain; yet to treat pain effectively it is necessary to have some concept of the suffering of the patient himself. Clinically pain and suffering are closely identified yet they are two distinct phenomena. The more severe the pain the more it is believed to cause suffering. There are however certain sorts of pain that are to some extent offset by parallel joy and fulfilment, as, for example, in childbirth. It is the perceived meaning of the pain which seems to influence the amount of medication required to control it. Cassel (1982) reports a patient who when she believed the pain in her leg was sciatica was able to control it with small doses of codeine, but as soon as she discovered that it was due to the spread of a malignant disease much greater amounts of narcotics were required for relief. He relates that 'patients can writhe in pain from kidney stones and by their own admission not be suffering, because they "know what it is"; they may also report considerable suffering from apparently minor discomfort when they do not know its source'. An expectant mother may be willing to deliver her baby without the aid of any analgesic, yet be most anxious to receive an oral narcotic for a comparatively mild post-partum pain. Older patients may view pain as a prelude to death. Toothache is more tolerable to bear than chest-pain, for it is realised that no matter how severe the ache in the tooth may be it does not endanger life.

It may be thought that pain is the least understood and the most neglected subject in medicine today. Much study of pain and its alleviation has however been undertaken over the past few decades and there is now an Intractable Pain Society of Great Britain and Ireland (founded in 1967), an International Association for the Study of Pain (1976), and also a bi-monthly journal, *Pain*, published by the association and exclusively devoted to the scientific study of pain. Pain clinics are now established in the United Kingdom and the United States with services varying from out-patient appointments to full in-patient care. More time and money than ever before has been devoted to research into the nature of pain and its relief, both in the clinic and in the laboratory.

Although most people very naturally regard it as an unpleasant sensation and something to be avoided at all costs, the value of pain cannot be disregarded. We have only to think of those people who have a congenital insensitivity to pain with a shortened life expectancy as a result. In its acute symptomatic form pain has a most important biological function. It serves as a protective mechanism for the body that occurs when tissues are damaged or threatened with damage, and so prompts the individual to react to prevent the damage. It is part of man's defences for survival. During an acute injury pain is the normal response to the disruption of healthy tissues, but continuation of pain beyond the period of healing indicates a persisting abnormality. The chronic pain state, however, has little or no positive biological value. The difference is emphasised by Bonica (1953) thus: 'In contrast in its chronic persistent form pain rarely, if ever, has a biologic function but is a malefic force that often imposes severe emotional, physical, economic and social stresses on the patient and on the family.'

As we all have to suffer pain from time to time we feel we know all about it, but the sensation of pain cannot be seen simply as the direct result of the stimulation of nerve endings of the pain fibres sending signals transmitted to the brain from the site of injury. It cannot be conceived solely as a simple cause-and-effect physical reaction, as something akin to the ringing telephone with the caller as the painful stimulus, the wires as peripheral nerves and the telephone receiver as the brain. Such a direct line theory, skin to brain, is far too simplistic for pain, as is proved when such examples of phantom limb, and primitive cultural practices such as '*couvade*' ('brood' or 'hatch') are considered. The *couvade* illustrates the impact that cultural values exercise on the degree of pain experienced in childbirth. In certain primitive cultures the 'woman who is going to give birth continues to work in the fields until the child is just about to be born. Her husband then gets into bed and groans as though he were in great pain while she bears the child. In more extreme cases, the husband stays in bed with the baby to recover from the terrible ordeal, and the mother almost immediately returns to attend the crops' (Melzack and Wall, 1965).

A phantom limb pain, sometimes experienced by a patient who has had a limb amputated (cf. Captain Ahab in Melville's *Moby Dick*), is believed to be the result of a pain memory after the original cause has been removed. Pain is felt in specific parts, such as the toe, and is usually described as a tingling or 'pins-and-needles' sensation. It may be episodic or a continuous dull presence, and is difficult to imagine by those who have not actually experienced it. The sensation has been described by Melzack (1973) as being so real that a person with an amputated arm would reach for a glass of water with that arm. He reports that the phantom can exist anywhere, so if a below-the-knee amputee were to rest the stump on a mattress, he or she might well feel that the lower leg and foot were inside the mattress. Melzack also relates that when Admiral Lord Nelson lost an arm in battle he wrote to a friend that he could still sense the missing arm and that he took this as evidence of his eternal soul. One patient in describing phantom limb pain after an above-knee amputation stated: 'I have gnawing pains as if crocodile teeth are biting into my ankle . . . I feel as though a chisel is turning round and round in my knee . . . my foot feels as though it has been jammed in a lift door.'

It is recognised that those who suffered prolonged pain in the affected limb prior to the amputation are more likely to develop phantom pain. It occurs in approximately 5 to 10 per cent of all amputees and is usually a subsequence of very painful and traumatic surgery. Generally it lasts in severity about three months but there are patients who experience such pain for a much longer period.

Pain is an extremely complex state with both physical and psychological factors involved. To do justice to the whole problem of pain means establishing a relationship with the total personality of the sufferer. It is 'whatever the patient says it is', states Sternbach (1974), 'and exists whenever he says it does. Real, psychogenic or imaginary, however meaningless it may appear to the doctor, each patient is zealously convinced of the validity and importance of his pain.'

Thus pain is not a simple physical sensation, but rather a dual phenomenon. It has two main components; *perception* and *reaction*. The pain perception threshold, which concerns the individual's interpretation of the meaning of the signals received in the brain, may be changed as a result of certain physical factors, as well as by attention or distraction. On the other hand the way in which an individual reacts to pain is far more complex. It is modulated by emotional, cultural and other factors; it varies considerably from one person to another, and also within the same person in different circumstances.

The perception of pain depends on the integrity of the nerve fibres that receive and transmit pain impulses and their central connections. There is a marked uniformity among people in the perception of pain. It has been stated that if a pin is pressed against the skin of 100 people, the amount of pressure necessary to cause pain would be practically similar in every case. Yet in such circumstances people's responses would vary widely. The reaction to pain has physiological manifestations, pallor, high blood pressure, muscle tension.

Loss of appetite, vomiting, nausea, irritability and restlessness are also not uncommon accompaniments. Behaviour responses will vary widely from one individual to another, and his physical condition, emotional state, the way in which he has been conditioned to respond to stressful situations, will all influence a patient's reaction.

Pain threshold, which is the stage at which a noxious stimulus is perceived as pain, is primarily physiological. Pain tolerance, which is the duration of time and the intensity of pain that a person accepts before making a verbal or overt pain response, is influenced by psychological and socio-cultural factors.

Patients who are hypochondriacal (see p. 13) and those who suffer from neurotic disorders have in general low pain thresholds. It has been found that in controlled laboratory experiments this perception threshold is remarkably similar in the majority of individuals in normal circumstances; that is, people subjected to an increasing amount of a painful stimulus, such as an increasing degree of heat applied to an area of the body, report feeling pain at almost exactly the same point of intensity of the stimulus. This threshold, however, may vary with a patient's physical condition or his emotional state at the time the pain is experienced. Factors which lower pain threshold include anxiety, fear, anger, depression, introversion, sympathy and analgesics. Men have slightly higher thresholds than women. Pain threshold seems to rise with age, for older people often bear pain more easily than the young whose previous experience has not prepared them for it. It will also vary according to mood, morale and meaning.

PSYCHOSOCIAL FACTORS

Merskey and Spear (1967) consider it is essential 'to evaluate both the pain experienced by the patient and the patient experiencing the pain'. The way in which a person perceives his pain and the way in which he reacts are influenced to a great extent by psychosocial factors. Not only personality attitudes to pain but also previous experiences and the present emotional and mental state of the patient must all be taken into account. From birth onwards each of us builds up a backcloth, as it were, of pain experiences, originating from the variety of peripheral painful stimulations which we experience through the course of our lives. It is for this reason that we vary in our personality characteristics and ways of handling the strains and stresses imposed by illness and pain. For example, in families that place a great deal of attention on pain, a child learns early that pain-related behaviours receive attention while other behaviours do not. Such an attitude can set a lifelong pattern of focusing on pain. Directly and indirectly the family environment affects the individual's ultimate response to pain.

Cultural, family and individual attitudes all colour concepts about pain and influence reactions. Each of us seems to have his or her unique 'pain personality'. Life experiences, sicknesses, pleasures and successes, miseries and failures, all form the nexus for illness. Experiences gathered during a lifetime are part of today as well as yesterday. A person who has never experienced severe pain may have little fear of it. Many a patient remarks, 'I never knew it was going to be as bad as this' or 'I never imagined anything could hurt so much'. Anger and resentment become common emotional reactions.

It is the 'whole person' in pain who has to be considered. Lériche's (1939) definition is a sound one: 'Physical pain is not a simple affair of an impulse travelling at a fixed rate along a nerve. It is the result of a conflict between a stimulus and the whole individual.' Pain is experienced by persons, not merely by bodies, for it is not pain per se which is to be treated but the person with the pain. What does his pain mean to him? How is it affecting him? It is no longer just a matter of having a hurt body, but he is 'a hurt body in totality', for all somatic pain has some psychological component. Pain is intimately related to both psyche and soma. The personal expectations of the patient about his pain have great influence, for people feel what they expect to feel. To one patient an injection may be an irritating pin-prick, to another it may become a frightening ordeal.

Pain as a sensation is closely associated with anxiety, worry, fear, anger, depression and other types of emotion. When a patient becomes fearful or anxious he tends to report that his pain is more intense; conversely when he becomes relaxed

10

and not anxious about the pain-producing stimulation he tends to report his pain as less intense. The total experience of pain involves a complex blending of unpleasant sensations with emotions.

A telling illustration of some of the psychological aspects of pain is found in the Lamentations of Jeremiah:

> Is it nothing to you, all ye that pass by? Behold, and see if there be any sorrow like unto my sorrow, which is done unto me, wherewith the Lord hath afflicted me in the day of his fierce anger. From above hath he sent fire into my bones . . . he hath made me desolate and faint all the day. (Lam. 1:12–13)

This passage may be taken as a reflection of the emotional distress caused by physical pain. Here too are the longing for attention and sympathy, and resentment and bitterness that others around do not fully appreciate what pain and suffering really mean. Again 'fire in my bones' may be an apt description of some types of pain (Merskey and Spear, 1967; Copp, 1985). It is interesting to note that the Hebrew word for pain (*makhov*) has been translated 'sorrow': 'is there any sorrow like my sorrow'. Pain seems to be equated with anguish.

For the anxious person pain will be greater because pain causes anxiety and anxiety in turn heightens pain. Anxiety and stress are seen as powerful potentiators of pain for they are the most common emotions aroused by acute pain, and depression, shame, guilt and anger can all influence the pain experience. All who minister to sick people are familiar with the fear and anxiety expressed in many a patient's face, for like pain itself these can reveal themselves in a variety of guises. There may be a dread that there is a sinister cause for pain: 'Is it cancer?' 'Can it be cured?'

There are people who seem prone to anxiety when having to face stressful situations and they are known to have an increased sensitivity to pain. For example, the torment of having to wait for the results of physical examinations and investigations give rise to anxiety. When an over-anxious person becomes ill he often has greater levels of pain than others who may have a calmer and more tranquil nature. One patient admirably expressed the vicious cycle of pain creating fear, which creates tension which intensifies pain, thus: 'Fear and pain became inseparable, and still are. I never had pain without fear, and fear intensified the pain. It was a vicious cycle that was difficult to break.' She went on to describe the inner tension: 'Inwardly I was screaming "be brave! be courageous!" outwardly I was crying and screaming pleas for help. I wanted so badly to release some of the feelings that were building up before they reached the explosion point. I was terrified!'

As well as of themselves being able to intensify pain, fear and anxiety can actually cause it in the first instance. It is inevitable that suffering necessarily forces the individual into a special position and leads to an excessive occupation with self. As Sternbach (1968, 1974) makes plain: 'All that is necessary for maximising pain responses is that anxiety responses also be great.' It has been said that fear of pain ranks second only to fear of death (Zborowski, 1969). Such anticipatory fears can often be more acute than the eventual pain itself. What such fear and anxiety of pain can mean to an individual has been well described by Louis Evely (1967):

> What is unbearable is not to suffer but to be afraid of suffering, to endure a precise pain, a definite loss, a hunger for something one knows – this is possible to bear. One can live with this pain. But in fear there is all the suffering in the world: to dread suffering is to suffer an infinite pain since one supposes it unbearable.

A person in pain has a myriad of thoughts and feelings. One patient wrote a journal composed of thoughts, perceptions, reactions, discoveries, and of letters addressed to 'Dear Pain', and the replies from 'Pain'. In one of the letters we read of Pain assuring her: 'Please try to accept me as I am in the present, not as I have been in the past or as you anticipate my being in the future' (Cady, 1976).

Fear and anxiety, those 'two grey sisters of pain', express two quite different psychological states. Fear is aroused by the knowledge that we are threatened by dangers whose effect can be foreseen. Such fear can be overcome and replaced by calmness and confidence. Anxiety, on the other hand, is the reaction to something vague and uncertain which can neither be fully understood nor appreciated, and consequently is only overcome with great difficulty.

Merskey (1967) studied the relationship between depression and pain. Persons who are constitutionally depressive personalities, and become depressed and down-hearted rather easily, have a tendency to feel more pain during illness than others who have a bright and cheerful disposition. Pain commonly occurs as a symptom in mental illness and particularly in depression. Depression is more often than not associated with chronic or prolonged pain (see p. 28) In the early stages of intractable pain anxiety is often experienced by patients, and later this can progress to feelings of depression *and* anxiety. The actual intensity of pain may not be affected by anxiety or depression, except to the extent that they precipitate physical changes, such as muscle tension, that may contribute noxious stimuli. Rather, it seems that anxiety and depression affect the patient's reaction to the pain or tolerance for pain – his outlook.

There are some individuals with marked hysterical personalities, who are inclined to make excessive demands for attention, exaggerate personal experiences, and play on people's emotions. They tolerate pain poorly and are inclined to be dramatic, highly extrovert and yet shallow in their affections. These tendencies can distort the presentation of a painful physical illness.

A common personality trait is that of hypochondriasis, and this can also colour or distort illness and patterns and responses to treatment. Certain people who have a rather morbid occupation with mental and bodily functions will consequently pay frequent visits to doctors. They will appear to be quite unconvinced about results of various investigations and become convinced that 'all is not well'. It has been estimated that about 10 per cent of regular attenders at general practitioners' surgeries are hypochondriacal and an unknown proportion of these will be preoccupied with pain. The major problem with such patients is determining whether their pain has a substantial or significant cause.

Engel (1959) notes that pain can never be neutral and refers to the fact that it may be associated with ideas of punishment, guilt, loss, threat and sexual gratification, and therefore with the emotions that may be expected to accompany such ideas, such as depression, anxiety and anger, which in turn frequently lead on to feelings of guilt and shame.

External circumstances may sometimes affect differences in behaviour and the variable meaning attached to pain-producing situations can greatly influence the degree and quality of pain experienced. It is often assumed that the greater the pain the more it is believed to cause suffering. Montaigne (1580) observed that *'nous sentons plus un coup de rasoir du chirurgien que dix coups d'espée en la chaleur du combat'* ('we feel a cut from the surgeon's scalpel more than ten blows of the sword in the heat of battle'). Guthrie (1827) in his study of gun-shot wounds in the Peninsular War noted that 'in two persons suffering apparently from the same kind of injury, and with the same detriment, one will writhe in agony, while the other will smile with contempt'.

Beecher (1956) in his famous study on the relationship of significance of wound to pain experience also showed how pain may be reduced in accordance with circumstances and expectations, and how external events around us affect both the severity of pain and behaviour associated with it. He observed how people who suffered similar wounds but under very different conditions experienced also very different degrees of pain. Much to his astonishment, of the soldiers severely wounded on the Anzio beach-head during the Second World War only one out of three taken into combat hospitals complained of sufficient pain to warrant morphine. They thought the war was over for them and that they would soon be well enough to be sent home. They were greatly relieved on being delivered from an area of danger.

With this group Beecher, when he returned to clinical practice as an anaesthetist, contrasted a series of civilians subjected to major surgery who had incisions similar to the wounds received by the soldiers. Of this latter group four out of five claimed they were in severe pain and asked for a morphine injection. The civilian's surgical operation was viewed as a 'depressing, calamitous event' by the majority. The pain arising from the surgeon's wounds was far greater than it was from the war wounds. The crucial difference appeared to lie in the significance of the two wounds and in the reaction of the patients to each.

The level of anxiety is important in considering the production of pain and the study concluded that:

> the common belief that wounds are inevitably associated with pain, and that the more extensive the wound the worse the pain, was not supported by observations made as carefully as possible in the combat zone ... there is no simple direct relationship between the wound per se and the pain experienced. Of great importance here is the significance of the wound ... in the wounded soldier (the response to injury) was relief, thankfulness at his escape alive from the battlefield, even euphoria; to the civilian, his major surgery was a depressing, calamitous event.

The wounds the soldiers suffered served to release them with honour from danger. There was no similar benefit to the civilians undergoing surgery, except that it was necessary to restore them, if possible, to normal health.

The lack of relationship between the severity of a surgical procedure and the pain response has also been confirmed in other studies. For example, Bruegel (1971) found that the amount of pain experienced was highest for persons who had undergone gastro-intestinal surgery and lowest for women undergoing Caesarean section – the gain of a baby is a much happier personal experience than the loss of a gall-bladder!

The author recalls hearing a London psychiatrist relate that many of the soldiers at Chelsea Barracks who were severely injured by long sharp nails during an IRA bombing attack did not feel their pain in the heat of the moment.

An Indian fakir is a striking example of internal pain control as he sits on his bed of nails. Some tribes in Africa and India are able to pierce their lips and cheeks with needles and stakes in ritualistic ceremonies and practices without appearing to experience pain. Football players and sportsmen and women in general can suffer quite severe injuries during a contest or event and yet not appear to notice any pain until afterwards, when the heat of the moment is past. A foremost pioneer in pain research relates of the time he landed a large salmon after a long and hearty struggle, only afterwards to find that he had a deep blood-dripping gash on his leg! These phenomena are of particular interest at the moment as our knowledge of endogenous opioids increases.

15

Religious attitudes also influence the pain response. Rather graphic examples may be found in the accounts of the early martyrs. In 'The martyrdom of Polycarp' (Ante-Nicene Library, vol I, ch. 2), for example, we read how some of the Christians:

> reached such a pitch of magnanimity, that not one of them let a sigh or a groan escape them; thus proving to us all that those holy martyrs of Christ, at the very time when they suffered such torments, were absent from the body, or rather, that the Lord then stood by them, and communed with them.

Huxley (1952) relates how those who were burnt at the stake for their religious convictions were often observed to experience what can only be described as 'ecstacy'. Their Christian faith and courage and the promise of future salvation all helped to transform an agonising situation into one of ecstacy. St Thomas Aquinas noted that 'the holy pleasure of contemplating divine things diminishes physical pain; and the martyrs suffered their pains more patiently because they were completely suffused with the love of God' (*Summa Theologica*, IV, Quaestio 15.5).

HOSPITAL STRESS AND PAIN

It has been previously noted that pain and anxiety are closely related phenomena, and for some persons the adjustment to the strange environment of a hospital can be a cause of much anxiety. Hospitalisation itself can induce significant stress. In his well-known study on the anxiety-creating effects of hospital admission Revans (1966) observes that 'hospitals are communities cradled in anxiety. Patients are anxious not only about their own health but about the welfare of their families . . . surgical patients in particular additionally face the direct physical threat of an operation.' Hospitalisation, as distinct from surgery, involves loss of independence, separation from family and unfamiliar routines and procedures, as well as the inevitable fears regarding health. Stability gives way to insecurity, and family and friends become 'visitors'.

Eight particular aspects of hospital life were found to be

especially stressful to the two hundred medical patients interviewed by Wilson-Barnett (1976, 1978, 1979). These were: being away from their family, absence from work, their condition or illness, the anticipation of a painful treatment, seeing a very ill patient, barium X-rays, using a bed-pan, and the night-time. All such factors, together with the patient's antecedent environment, may influence the pain experience. There is a tendency among some patients to be apprehensive and worried about the possibility of mistakes and/or neglect during hospitalisation (Tagliacozzo and Mauksch, 1972). Lack of privacy may be another cause of anxiety and a contributory factor in the perception of pain. Mumford and Skipper (1967) indicate the concern for the outcome when new patients are 'propelled almost immediately into contact that is intimate in nature, crucial in outcome'.

Commenting on the patient's admission to a new environment, Gillis (1962) describes a hospital as a most inappropriate place in which to be ill. At home the person is 'special', in hospital he becomes 'ordinary': at home he may be the most sick member of the family, in hospital he may find himself the most healthy patient of the ward. Such experiences are verbalised with difficulty and are more readily studied through their non-verbal manifestations. Studies reveal that patients especially vulnerable to strong anxiety feelings include those with characteristically high levels of anxiety and depression 'proneness', females under forty years of age, those who have not been in hospital before, those admitted for a series of special tests, and those with 'infective' or 'undiagnosed' illnesses. The following statements by patients are indicative of some of the feelings experienced: 'I feel all tied up inside'; 'They don't seem to tell you anything'; 'I haven't had any results from the tests yet and I'm terrified'; 'I was suddenly taken off to be X-rayed – no one told me why'; 'I don't think they are telling me the truth.'

Illness to the patient means much more than a mere constellation of symptoms: it is a period in which his emotional, social and economic securities are threatened. Alongside his physical distress will be mental and emotional stress and he soon becomes reminded of both his somatic and his psychological fallibilities. A study by Lucente and Fleck

17

(1972) of hospitalisation anxiety among 408 medical and surgical patients made the following observations:

1. *Age*. Anxiety decreased as age increased.
2. *Religion*. Roman Catholic patients were generally more anxious than others.
3. *Sex*. Female patients were generally more anxious than male patients.
4. *Service* to which admitted. Gynaecological and orthopaedic patients showed higher levels of anxiety than general surgical patients.

It is interesting to note that they found no consistent correlation between the patient's anxiety level and the type of illness. Malignancy was the only exception. Cancer patients tended to be more anxious than other patients. Other important aspects to be considered are the patient's antecedent environment (his home and all from which he is separated), hospital characteristics (the physician-patient relationship may produce or allay anxiety or stress, communication being the central issue), the nature of the illness (worries, fears, anxieties all spring into awareness), and the person who is the patient (the most variable factor of all four aspects, for much depends upon the patient's personality and background in determining his predisposition to the experience of anxiety, stress and fear).

INFORMATION

Hayward (1975) has shown how information can be a prescription against pain; how pain is influenced by anxiety, and that in turn anxiety is influenced by information about future events. Lack of information, acting via the medium of increased anxiety, can occasion more pain and suffering in postoperative patients than perhaps need be the case. It must not be overlooked, however, that some patients may not always hear what is being said to them on account of the very presence of pain.

In a study carried out by Cartwright (1964) in twelve randomly selected districts in England and Wales, over a hundred former hospital patients were interviewed in their homes. Of these, 61 per cent said that they had experienced some difficulty in obtaining information while they were in hospital, and 29 per cent voiced dissatisfaction. Patients seem to establish a better rapport with physicians in smaller hospitals than in large teaching hospitals. 'Medicine seems curiously inept in its communication with its customers' (*BMJ*, 1976). A DHSS Report (1963) which dealt with the subject of communication between doctors, nurses and patients, indicated that what seems to the doctor or nurse to be simple straightforward information may not be understood or absorbed even by the intelligent layman. Lack of information was also reported by 95 out of 110 patients in a study of patient satisfaction undertaken by the King Edward's Hospital Fund (1969). Barnes (1961) viewed the hospital as job or task-orientated, rather than patient orientated, and so communication within the hospital becomes a major problem. Such weaknesses have been commented upon in the writings of Solzhenitsyn (*Cancer Ward*, 1971) and Illich (*Medical Nemesis*, 1975) and such apprehension can have a detrimental effect upon the patient's pain experience.

There is evidence too to prove that some patients who are worried and tense before undergoing surgery take longer to recover and experience more pain than patients who have been given adequate information.

There are some who have rather vivid memories of previous operations when anaesthesia was induced using a mask, and for them modern anaesthetic procedures can still become 'an unnatural sleep, a kind of death'. Consequently many will express more fear of anaesthesia than about the operation itself. There are studies which show that stress before surgery is positively related to discomfort and pain experienced postoperatively. Least postoperative disturbance and pain were shown by those patients who were *moderately* fearful before their operation. They recognised the threat, and thus had the opportunity and incentive to prepare themselves for it psychologically, but were not so vigilant to threat that they were overwhelmed by it (Janis, 1958, 1971).

The meaning of the operation has an influence in determining the emotions of the patient. Where patients have received information with reassurance regarding surgery and coping devices, such as calming self-talk, they seem to have the highest tolerance of pain, least quantity of analgesic and earliest ambulation and discharge. The reflection of one patient who suffered severe postoperative pain illustrates how important such preparatory information is:

> I'd have given anything if someone had said to me the night before the operation: 'You're going to experience pain like you've never felt before, but we are here to help you.' I doubt that this would have frightened me too much since a description of pain was what I was expecting intellectually. But just to have known that someone understood how rough it was going to be and cared enough to promise their support would have meant so much.

In one study (Egbert et al., 1964) ninety-seven special-care patients were told what to expect after their surgery, and were shown how to relax and how to move to be more comfortable during the initial postoperative period. It was found that the postoperative requirement was halved compared with that of the control group and patients were ready for discharge three days earlier.

CULTURAL ASPECTS

It is interesting to note that major cultural differences determine attitudes towards and reactions to pain, although the ability to experience pain in response to noxious stimuli differs little between races. Members of various cultures may react differently in terms of their manifest behaviour towards various pain experiences and this behaviour is often dictated by the culture which provides specific norms according to the age, sex and social position of the individual. It is suggested that rather than the perception of intensity of the stimuli, it is cultural origin which influences our reaction to painful stimuli. Zborowski (1969) studied four readily identifiable groups in the USA and was able to find significant differences between cultural groups including Italians and Jews, and Irish and third-generation Americans. He found that Italians and Jews tended to manifest similar behaviour in terms of their reactions to pain. They felt free to talk about their pain, complain about it and manifest their suffering by groaning, moaning, and crying. They were not ashamed of these expressions, and expected a great deal of assistance and sympathy from others. The 'Old American', who is closely akin to the average Briton, tried to avoid being a nuisance, was phlegmatic and matter of fact about pain. They were future-orientated and tended to withdraw socially, and adopted an uncomplaining manner with few verbal or physical expressions of pain. The Irish patients were reluctant to discuss their pain and believed that they were not expected to share their troubles with anyone. Identical findings were reported in a later study by Sternbach and Tursky (1965) which looked at the ethnic differences among Yankees (that is, 'Old Amercians' or Protestants of British descent), Irish, Jewish and Italian housewives.

Zborowski found the age variable important in three areas: older patients were more prone to show pain than hide it; older patients valued the doctor's personality above his skills, and middle-aged patients tended to delay the least in consulting a doctor. Woodrow et al. (1972) observed that generally pain tolerance decreased with age, men tolerate more pain than women, and whites tolerate more pain than orientals, while blacks occupy an intermediate position.

Severity of pain and associated behaviour is determined to a large extent by the interaction of personality and environmental factors. In our western culture it is easier for women to display pain perception than men since this is the recognised norm. Much of the behaviour we express when in pain has been learnt from various models of behaviour in our early childhood, usually from our parents and/or sick relations. The governing factor seems to be the level of approval given in a particular culture for the public expression of pain and emotion.

Aristotle   *Nicomathean Ethics*, Bk. II, tr. D. Ross. OUP, London 1954; *Treatise on the Principles of Life*, Eng. tr. W. A. Hammond, Bk. II, ch. 6; Bk. III, ch. 1.

Barnes, E. *People in Hospital*. Macmillan, London 1961.

Beecher, H. K. 'Relationship of significance of wound to pain experienced', *J. Amer. Medical Assoc.*, 161:17 (1956), pp. 1609–12.
Measurement of Subjective Responses. OUP, London 1959.

Bonica, J. J. *The Management of Pain*. Lea & Febiger, Philadelphia 1953.
(ed.) *Advances in Neurology*, vol IV. Raven Press, New York 1974.
'Introduction to Symposium on Pain' *Arch. Surg.*, 112 (June 1977).

British Medical Journal Qu. *Guardian*, 20 May 1976, in *BMJ*, 1 (1976), p. 1362.

Bruegel, M. A. 'Relationship of preoperative anxiety to perception of postoperative pain', *Nurs. Res.* 20:26 (1971).

Cady, J. W. 'Dear Pain', *Amer. J. Nursing* (June 1976), pp. 950–1.

Cartwright, A. *Human relations and Hospital Care*. Routledge & Kegan Paul, London 1964.

Cassel, E. J. 'The nature of suffering and the goals of medicine', *New Eng. J. Med.* (18 March 1982), pp. 639–45.

Copp, L. A. 'The spectrum of suffering', *Amer. J. Nursing*, 74:3 (1974), pp. 491–5.
(ed.) *Recent Advances in Nursing: perspectives on pain*. Churchill Livingstone, Edinburgh 1985.

DHSS *Report . . . on communication between Doctors, Nurses and Patients*, Dept Health & Soc. Sec. HMSO, London 1963.

Egbert, L. D. et al. 'Reduction of post-operative pain by encouragement and instruction of patients', *New Eng. J. Med.*, 270 (1964), pp. 823–7.

Engel, G. L. ' "Psychogenic" pain and the pain-prone patient' *Amer. J. Med*, 26 (1959), pp. 899–918.

Evely, L. *Suffering*. Burns & Oates; and Herder & Herder, London 1967.

Gillis, L. *Human Behaviour in Illness*. Faber, London 1962.

Guthrie, G. J.   *A Treatise on Gunshot Wounds*. London 1827.

Hayward, J.   'Pain: psychological and social aspects', *Nursing*, 1 (1980), pp. 21–7.
Information: A Prescription against Pain: The study of nursing care. Research Project, ser. 2, No. 5 (RCN, London 1975).

Hick, J.   *Evil and the God of Love*. Fontana Lib. of Theology and Philosophy, London 1968.

Huxley, A.   *The Devils of Loudon*. Harper, NY 1952.

Janis, I. L.   *Psychological Stress*. Wiley, New York 1958.
Stress and Frustration. Harcourt, Brace & Jovanovich, New York 1971.

King Edward's Hospital Fund   *Patients and their Hospitals*. King Edward's Hospital Fund for London 1969.

Lériche, R.   *The Surgery of Pain*, tr. and ed. Archibald Young. Bailliere, Tindall & Cox, London 1939.

Lewis, C. S.   *The Problem of Pain*. Fontana, London 1940.

Lewis, T.   *Pain*. Macmillan, New York 1942.

Locke, J.   *Essay Concerning Human Understanding*. 1690.

Lucente, F. E. and Fleck, S.   'A study of hospitalization anxiety in 408 medical and surgical patients', *Psychosom. Med.*, 34 (1972), pp. 304–12.

Melzack, R.   *The Puzzle of Pain*. Penguin, London 1973.

Melzack, R., and Torgerson, W. S.   'On the language of pain', *Anesthesiology*, 34:50 (1971).

Melzack, R., and Wall, P. D.   'Pain mechanisms: A new theory', *Science*, 150 (1965), pp. 971–9.
The Challenge of Pain. Penguin, London 1982.
The Textbook of Pain. Churchill Livingstone, Edinburgh 1984.

Merskey, H.   'Psychological aspects of pain', *Postgrad. Med. J.*, 44 (1967), p. 297.

Merskey, H., and Spear, F. G.   *Pain: psychological and psychiatric aspects*. Bailliere, Tindall & Cassell, London 1967.

Mumford, E., and Skipper, J. K.   *Sociology in Hospital Care*. Harper & Row, New York 1967.

Revans, R. W.   *Standards for Morale*. OUP, London 1966.

Sternbach, R. A.   'Congenital insensitivity to pain: a critique', *Psychol. Bulletin*, 60 (1963), pp. 252–64.
Pain: a psycho physiological analysis. Academic Press, New York 1968.

23

Sternbach, R. A.	(ed.) *The Psychology of Pain*. Raven Press, New York 1978. *Pain Patients: traits and treatment*. Academic Press, New York 1974.
Sternbach, R. A., and Tursky, B.	'Ethnic differences among housewives in psychophysical and skin potential to electric shock', *Psychophysiology*, 1 (1965), pp. 241–6.
Tagliacozzo, D. L., and Mauksch, H. D.	'The patient's view of the patient's role', in *Patients, Physicians and Illness*, ed. E. C. Jaco. Free Press, New York (1972), pp. 162–75.
Wilson-Barnett, J.	'Patients' emotional reactions to hospitalization: an explanatory study', *J. Adv. N.*, 1 (1976), pp. 351–8. 'Factors influencing patients' emotional reactions to hospitalization', *J. Adv. N.*, 3 (1978), pp. 221–9. *Stress in Hospital: Patients' Psychological Reaction to Illness & Health Care*. Churchill Livingstone, Edinburgh 1979. 'Interventions to alleviate patients' stress: a review', *J. Psychosomatic Res.*, 28:1 (1984), pp. 63–72.
Woodrow, K. M., et al.	'Pain differences according to age, sex, and race', *Psychom. Med.*, 34 (1972), pp. 548–56.
Woolf, V.	'On being ill', in *The Moment and Other Essays* (Harcourt, Brace, New York 1948), pp. 9–23.
Zborowski, M.	'Cultural components in response to pain', *J. Social Issues*, 8 (1952), pp. 16–30. *People in Pain*. Jossey-Bass, San Francisco 1969.

2

Variety of Pain

But pain is perfect miserie, the worst of evils, and excessive, overturnes all patience.

John Milton, *Paradise Lost*, Bk 6

Joy and pain like other simple ideas cannot be described or their names defined . . . we get to know them only by experience.

John Locke (1690)

To assess a subjective event experienced by someone else is an extremely difficult task. The words of Laing (1975) ring true: 'I cannot experience your experience. You cannot experience my experience. We are both invisible men. All men are invisible to one another.' We cannot take a sample of pain and analyse it. To complicate the issue further, there is a wide variation in how people experience pain, including the fact that the same person may react to pain differently at different times. No observer however experienced can ever measure another person's pain, the severity of which can be known only to the sufferer concerned.

The famous surgeon René Lériche (1939) outlined the problem graphically:

What we have not personally experienced, it is not easy for us to realise, and what we are told by those who suffer appeals only to our imagination. The victims of pain may give very imperfect descriptions of what they feel . . . for the moment we accept their description, but we do not realise the duration of this hell on earth, and if we try to get them to be more precise, our patients do not succeed in going beyond these few words . . . It is vain for you to

25

examine the part, to touch it with your fingers. There is nothing to be seen. There is nothing for you to feel, for the pain is not in any respect objective. As regards pain, a subjective phenomenon, the healthy person does not get beyond the threshold of the unknowable.

THE ASSESSMENT OF PAIN

While pain cannot be measured, attempts to assess it are most essential and are vital tasks for all who have to minister, for they affect their ability to understand the basic concepts of pain and to produce a proper clinical diagnosis and relevant treatment.

Apart from the physiological responses which frequently occur with patients in severe acute pain when the sympathetic nervous system is activated and the release of adrenalin produces increased pulse, increased respiration and blood pressure, perspiration, dilated pupils, pallor, nausea and muscle tension, there are other signals to be taken into account. Various persons speak of suffering not only by their moans or cries but also with their bodies. McCaffery (1972) has identified various types of body movements which may be indicative of distress and discomfort: immobilisation which helps to minimise pain, purposeless movement (tossing in bed, kicking, in severe pain), protective, and rubbing and rhythmic movements. Again facial expressions such as wrinkled forehead, biting of the lower lip, widely opened or tightly closed eyes and clenched teeth, or other facial grimaces, may be evidence of pain.

Some studies suggest that a verbal statement from the patient is generally the most informative measure concerning pain. In other words it is what the individual says it is, a unique, personal and subjective state. 'The simplest and most reliable index of pain', states Lasagna (1958), 'is the patient's verbal report.' Importance should always be attached to the patient's own perception of his pain. Melzack and Torgerson (1971) identified ninety-two words used to describe pain. The patient's task is to choose the words which most closely describe his pain at the time. Many patients express satisfaction at being given the opportunity to convey the exact nature of their pain. As Gracely (1979) comments: 'Man's unique verbal abilities open a window to private experience and only through such an experience is pain defined.' The description patients give to their experience can afford reliable clues to the possible cause of their pain. Melzack and Torgerson's study of the language of pain developed a list of pain 'descriptors' which formed three major categories: sensory (throbbing, burning, cramping, and so on); affective (sickening, terrifying, blinding); and evaluative (annoying, miserable, unbearable). It was observed that people from widely divergent backgrounds tend to use the same comparisons to familiar objects, such as 'like a knife' or 'hammers pounding inside the head', to describe different sorts of headache. Adjectives so used – 'dull', 'sharp', 'aching', 'throbbing', 'burning', 'tightening' – are all of some importance and of much diagnostic value.

Although these descriptions of pain are easily identified and appropriate care can be planned, for patients who do not admit to discomfort other clues must be sought in the subtle behaviour they present. It is often helpful to patients who cannot find the right words to describe their pain to point to words and numbers. Confusion can easily arise in questioning patients, if the term 'pain' means one thing to a doctor or nurse, while to the patient it means something else. Should a patient respond negatively to the question it should not be taken for granted therefore that he is not in pain. Affect changes which can signify pain include excitement, irritability, depression, unusual quietness, withdrawal or behaviour reversals such as hostility from an ordinarily calm person. The importance of forestalling the evolution of unacceptable pain cannot be over-emphasised.

There are a number of patients who seem reluctant to confess they are in pain. Of seventy-two patients studied by Jacox and Stewart (1973) approximately two-thirds stated that they tried to remain calm and did not want to show they were in pain.

ACUTE PAIN

Clinically pain is frequently divided into two major groups which are seen as distinct entities – *acute* and *chronic*. Acute pain is relatively short-lived and frequently adequately dealt with. It normally follows trauma and is experienced by everyone at some stage or other in their lives. It can range from relatively minor (toothache, headache, bruise or sprain) to major (myocardial infarction and postoperative). It has a beginning and an end and is readily understood by patients, families, medical and nursing staff, and the lay public. It is short-term and has a known, treatable cause or a defined course of illness.

The overall pattern of acute pain is one of emergency response, the fight or flight reaction. Such short duration discomfort raises the level of anxiety and fear, with preoccupation with the cause of the pain and consequences. Acute pain is normally viewed positively as a warning signal which draws attention to injury or illness. When appropriate action is taken acute pain can be remedied. One of the major advances has been the recognition of the difference between acute and chronic pain.

CHRONIC PAIN

Chronic, or better, 'intractable' pain presents a rather different picture. In contrast to acute pain, chronic persistent pain has no biological value, and is a most disabling disease. Although equally well recognised it is rather poorly understood. It can become a medical problem in its own right (Bonica, 1973). Chronic pain is to be seen, too, as a major social problem, for the sufferer lives in a complex system involving other people – family, friends, physicians and carers. Fiendishly, uselessly, pain signals keep firing in the nervous system for weeks, months, even years.

We can attempt to avoid acute pain and distance ourselves psychologically where the stimulus is external, but:

with chronic or inner pains there is no object to regard, or to avoid. The pain overwhelms us. We cannot place a psychological distance between ourselves and the hurt, and we are not merely threatened, but invaded and occupied. It is not any longer a matter of *having* a body that has a hurt member, but we *are* a body that is almost entirely pain. (Sternbach, 1968)

Saunders (1970) warns that chronic pain is not a mere 'extention in time of acute pain'. There is a qualitative difference; it affects the whole person, psychologically, physiologically, emotionally and spiritually. Therapies that are effective in the treatment of acute pain are frequently ineffective and often counter-productive when used in the patient who suffers from chronic pain. Chronic pain can be characterised as a vicious circle with no set time limit. Melzack (1973) observes that the fearful anticipation of its perpetration leads to anxiety, depression and insomnia which in turn accentuate the physical component of the pain. Chronic pain, in contrast to acute, is seen by Twycross (1984) as a *situation* rather than an *event*. It is impossible to predict when it will end; it often gets worse rather than better; it lacks positive meaning, and it frequently expands to occupy the patient's whole attention and isolates him from the world around him. It is hardly ever anticipated, is often poorly controlled, and has been defined as 'a circular continuum of aching to agony'. Chronic pain has been well described in a poem by Emily Dickinson (c. 1862):

> Pain – has an element of blank –
> It cannot recollect
> When it begun – or if there were
> A time when it was not –

The dominant emotions associated with chronic pain are depression and anger, and they have a substantial impact on the psychological and social well-being of the patient. The chronically ill patient feels invaded, trapped and fully occupied by his pain. His life seems to centre round home, doctor's surgery and hospital out-patients department. It has been noted by McCaffery (1983) how, in their search for remedies, those in chronic pain can readily develop the 'Naaman's syndrome'; that which is readily to hand becomes devalued and the doctor's waiting-room as unattractive as the muddy

Jordan! 'Are not Abana and Pharpar, rivers of Damascus, better than all the waters of Israel? May I not wash in them, and be clean? So he turned and went away in a rage' (2 Kings 5:12). As the pain seems to serve no biologically useful purpose, and at times can be so terrible, many people would sooner die than live with it. They are beset by a sense of helplessness and meaninglessness, and consequently suicide is not uncommon. One patient described her chronic intractable pain as 'a world of living hell', and reflected: 'After a few years, persons with pain do not fear death: what they fear is living. Some even envy patients with terminal cancer because they at least will die: the painridden individual must live. A longer life only means more pain and destruction.' Sternbach (1974) in describing the seeming endlessness of chronic suffering recalls the remark of one of his patients: 'It's always three o'clock in the morning.' Such patients never feel rested, and become worn down, worn out and exhausted.

The unhappy state of chronic pain has been called the 'terrible triad' of suffering, sleeplessness, and sadness, a calamity that is as hard on the family as it is on the victim. Meinhart and McCaffery (1983) relate that one patient in chronic pain described how his body formed a prison around the person he really was. He wanted to laugh, enjoy life and engage in all his previous activities but his pain acted like the prison walls, keeping him from stepping out into his former life. Another patient of thirty-one years of age said his chronic pain made him feel like an old man.

Describing the world of the patient in chronic pain, LeShan (1964) perceives a similarity to the universe of the nightmare. He outlines the structural components of a terror dream and relates them to the person in a chronic condition: terrible things are being done to him and worse are threatened: others, or outside forces, are in control and the will is helpless: there is no time limit set, and no one cannot predict when it will be over. The person in chronic pain is in the same situation: terrible things are being done to him and he does not know if worse will happen: he has no control and is helpless to take effective action: no time limit is given. 'The patient lives during the waking state in the cosmos of the nightmare.'

PSYCHOSOCIAL EFFECTS OF CHRONIC PAIN

The experience of severe chronic pain may involve physical (the pathological process), psychological (anxiety and depression), and social dimensions (loneliness and hostility). If often leads to a gradual disintegration of personality where formerly the individual was entirely normal and contented with his lot. The psychosocial impact of life with chronic pain appears more directly related to how such inhibitions of functioning and changes of life-style are perceived by the individual concerned. Much will depend on how he has handled adaptations and stresses of life prior to the onset of his pain. Family relationships may become disrupted and social activities restricted. Role reversal *vis-à-vis* employment often aggravates an already drastic emotional alteration. Frequent visits to hospital or out-patient clinics, when necessary, are apt to disrupt family life and often family finances. Members of the family encounter depression, anxiety, loss of self-esteem and increased dependency. Where there are young children they may face emotional distancing from the chronic pain patient as he becomes increasingly introverted and preoccupied with his own condition. The whole emotional stability of the household may possibly fluctuate from day to day, being dependent upon the patient's level of pain.

Many people in chronic pain become uncharacteristically rude or openly aggressive, and anger and hostility are projected on those offering guidance and relief. This in turn can isolate the patient and alienate the affection and understanding of family, friends and even medical and nursing staff. There may already exist family stresses, with heavy and unnecessary demands made on those around, the family kept 'to heel and order'. Understandably the search for an 'answer' or a remedy becomes paramount, and there is often a resource to fringe medicine, 'faith-healers', or any agency that promises quick and permanent 'cures'.

A study undertaken by Rowat (1983) revealed that over 75 per cent of spouses considered that their marital relationships were affected by the chronic pain condition of their partner. 'I didn't get married to be alone, now that I am alone I feel to a certain extent separated from my wife by this experience', was a typical reaction. The family becomes restricted socially and members see themselves faced with 'having to live with it', as feelings of uncertainty and helplessness blur the reality of the present and the future. Such questions arise as: How do I act: sympathetic or firm? Do I ignore him? How will my behaviour affect his pain? (Rowat, 1983).

There is great need for the family itself to be seen as a unit of care, and not solely the individual suffering in isolation. Ideally all should be under the total management of the health team. Such a model was advocated by Geyman (1977): 'There is an important conceptual and practical difference between caring for the individual in the context of the family and caring for the family itself as the patient.'

It is this particular group of chronically ill patients that challenges physicians in their management of pain, for chronic pain remains an enigma that can mystify even the most experienced clinician. Chronic pain seems to confer no clear biological service, nor is it usually ennobling or uplifting (Sternbach, 1974). To the patient it seems meaningless as well as endless. The consequences of chronic pain are far-reaching and must be considered in both physical and emotional terms. It is a problem which is on the increase for people are now living longer with chronic diseases and other disorders associated with pain.

POSTOPERATIVE PAIN

More attention has recently been given to the widespread problem of postoperative pain. Studies show that among a large number of postoperative patients, one third do not complain of postoperative pain, one third complain of mild to moderate pain, and the other third complain of severe pain. Bonica (1983) estimates that of patients who undergo major surgery some 5 to 20 per cent suffer minimal pain, 25 to 40 per cent endure moderate pain, and the remaining 25 to 40 per cent experience severe pain. The amount of pain will of course vary greatly dependent upon the site and extent of the surgery, but also the sex, age, personality and emotional status of the patient will all exert their influence. Young patients seem to bear postoperative pain well while the elderly generally react less well. The sort of incision that involves severing or damaging many nerves obviously produces more pain than those involving only a few nerves. It has already been noted how fear and anxiety can increase the probability of postoperative pain and discomfort when they are disproportionate to the severity of the surgery (Janis, 1958). Most patients seem to fear the degree of pain and discomfort they are likely to suffer as well as the anxiety and uncertainty as to what might happen to them. Often the content of their fear is imagined and fantasised. Wilson-Barnett (1979) has shown that many worry about themselves, about being 'cut', about dying, about change in their appearance and body, and about losing control of their bodily functions and consciousness. Other pain-related concerns will be: Will I be able to stand the pain? What will it be like? Will I be given something to ease the pain?

Pain being the very private experience it is can of course vary greatly, but postoperatively it is normally worst during the first forty-eight hours. It always seems worse and more intolerable at night and in the small hours of the morning. Night is a time of isolation when fears of helplessness are paramount, when sounds are muted, and verbal and aural stimulation diminished. There is the added fear of disturbing others or of appearing to be 'a nuisance'. 'I found pain and time, especially at night, to be bad companions', wrote one former patient after his operation. Pain postoperatively is probably more severe after upper abdominal and thoracic incisions, and less severe after surgery on the lower abdomen, head and neck. It usually consists of a dull constant ache but any movement or coughing can produce sharp and severe pain.

In one study undertaken by Loan and Morrison (1976), it was found that out of one thousand patients undergoing general surgical or urological operations 36 per cent required no analgesic drug postoperatively. Predisposing factors such as personality type, intelligence level, social class, personal traits, family background, may account for such different attitudes and psychological variables:

Most experienced clinicians have noticed the dramatic change that occurs in some patients recuperating from

33

surgery when the spouse visits. A stoic, composed individual bearing up well under the pain of a major incision may change in an instant to a weeping, moaning, and altogether pathetic character when the spouse appears at the bedside. If patient and spouse have a dependence-nurturance relationship pain is exaggerated when the spouse is present. If instead the spouse expects stoicism and courage, the patient may appear to suffer less in his or her presence. (Chapman, 1985).

Situational factors also have a part to play, for where there have been preparation, encouragement and information postoperative pain and discomfort have been reduced. In one day-care unit patients awaiting hernia repair are lent a medical cassette tape which explains the condition, its surgical repair and the postoperative care (Baskerville et al., 1985). The information is disseminated not only to the patient but to his family. All but 2 per cent of the patients found the tape beneficial and noted that such information and preparation alleviated much of their own and their relatives' anxiety.

PSYCHOGENIC PAIN

There are conditions in which an individual will complain of pain but no medical evidence of tissue damage or nerve irritation can be found. Such a person is then said to be having psychogenic pain, the implication being that the primary cause is psychological; the person is presumed to be in pain because he needs or wants it. Breuer and Freud, in their *Studies on Hysteria* (1895), published detailed case-histories demonstrating pain convincingly as a psychological manifestation. There is usually a general reluctance on the patient's part to acknowledge that pain can be psychologically induced, for such a concept makes little sense to the person experiencing it. It is far easier, for example, to say, 'I have a pain in my stomach', than 'I am suffering from a broken heart'. Whether the cause is primarily physical or mainly psychological it is essential to explain that there is often no marked difference in the pain felt. There is no such thing as 'imaginary' pain. Psychogenic pain is not necessarily experienced differently from pain of an organic origin.

So many sufferers fear being branded as 'malingerers', or being put off with 'it's all in the mind' attitudes. It is therefore extremely important to reserve the title 'psychogenic' for pain that has no organic origin and patients who have a definite psychological history which involves them in the need to express emotional problems in terms of pain. We should not think of a clear dichotomy between psychogenic and organic pain, for there is probably no pain that human beings suffer that is purely organic or strictly functional. It is an extremely difficult task to differentiate between psychogenic and somatogenic pain.

The following characteristics of pain of psychogenic origin have been classified by Merskey (1968):

1. It does not arouse the patient from sleep;
2. it is usually continuous from day to day, except at night, or else lasts for upwards of one hour;
3. it is commonest in the form of headaches, and often involves more than one area of the body;
4. the most common associated personality traits include hostility, resentment, and guilt;
5. it may respond to psychiatric treatment.

Most localised pain sensations are the result of both physical and mental aspects, although a different balance will be seen in different patients. It seems more useful to think of a pain continuum in which psychological factors play a greater or lesser role.

TRANSACTIONAL ASPECTS

Psychogenic pain patients are usually studied by psychologists and psychiatrists, to whom they are referred when their doctors are unable to find adequate physical explanations for the condition. In the psychological overplay there are associated symbolic meanings; and an analysis of behaviour patterns has been studied by Szaz (1957) and Engel (1959). For example, complaints of pain may be associated with the

35

concept of punishment; with strong feelings of guilt and shame over comparatively petty misdemeanours; or based on fact or fantasy. Pain might be used to manipulate emotional reactions and situations to the sufferer's advantage, and guilt provoked among his family or friends. Patients may become excessively demanding and dependent or attempt to fulfil needs which they feel themselves helpless to meet.

It was Szaz (1957) who used the term 'painmanship' to describe the interaction which occurs between pain patients and their physicians. On the one hand the doctor is anxious to diagnose the cause of the pain and identify its source and relieve the suffering, while on the other the patient is equally keen to be seen and identified as a painful suffering person with pain which cannot be diagnosed and suffering which cannot be relieved. It becomes extremely difficult for the physician to differentiate between the patient who really wants relief, and the one who demands it but does not intend to get well.

Szaz noted the communicative aspect and symbolic meaning of pain. The patient is attempting to say something other than registering the fact that he is in pain. Such a communicative aspect may include an allegation of injustice, rejection, or revenge. 'See how much I am suffering.' 'I hope you realise what you have done to me in the past.' 'Think of what you are doing to me now.' Those who have been deprived of sympathy in the past may in effect be saying: 'I want you to take pity on me. Stay with me. Don't ever leave me.' The relief of self-guilt is often sought in expressions of aggression, the avoidance of work in expressions of anxiety and apprehension.

Sternbach (1974) describes as 'pain-games' the various forms of behaviour and interactions of patients with chronic pain from benign disorders towards family, friends, physicians and others. Berne, in *Games that People Play* (1966), described the 'pain-games' that a number of chronic pain sufferers indulged in to convince their doctors of the severity of their complaints, which never seemed able to be relieved. In spite of all reassurances from the doctor symptoms are apt to become worse. The clinical picture seems dominated by pain and suffering. Sternbach sees that certain themes and patterns recur between many patients and the persons who are important to them. For example, there is the 'home-tyrant' who is determined to get his own way, and uses his pain to excuse himself from responsibilities and yet save face. 'Don't keep bothering me now, my back is bad!' 'I would gladly do it but I've got a splitting headache at the moment.' The pain serves as an excuse with honour. The word 'can't' becomes inaccurate; what is really meant is 'don't want to'. Through such attitudes others are found to do things for him, and he receives what he wants – attention, sympathy, tender loving care. The 'confounder' plays the game of gaining full attention from various doctors by complaining of pain. The more specialised and well-known the doctor the better. Each doctor gets defeated in the end: the emotional needs of the patient for attention are fulfilled, and often the need for punishment is attained through the form of unpleasant investigation.

Engel (1959) suggested that there are certain individuals, whom he calls 'pain-prone', for whom the presence of pain is essential for the prevention or relief of emotional turmoil. They appreciate the role of penitence, atonement, self-denial, and self-deprecation as means of self-inflicted punishment to ease their feelings of guilt. Many such patients are chronically depressive, have very little joy and no enthusiasm for life. They are inclined to drift into relationships in which they get hurt or humiliated; and conspicuously fail to exploit situations which would normally lead to success and happiness. When success seems imminent a painful symptom often develops. Such behaviour fulfils their need to be seen as 'a martyr' who tolerates suffering, and pain and discomfort become unconscious sources of gratification. A history of suffering, punishment and defeat has often played an important role in early family relationships and a pattern of suffering established in childhood.

Psychogenic patients seem to be neurotically depressed and hypochondriacal. More women than men suffer psychogenic pain which appears to parallel the greater incidence of neurotic disorders among them. It is important to be reminded that it is only a small percentage of patients who react in this way compared to the vast numbers of those who have various pain problems. They are usually very rare, very sensitive individuals who can experience pain by merely thinking certain thoughts, or by imagining certain situations, and represent an abnormal type of personality development.

TERMINAL PAIN

Terminal pain, which tends to be chronic, is any sort of pain being experienced by a dying patient. Saunders (1967) developed the concept of 'total pain' to cover the psychological, financial, interpersonal and spiritual, as well as physical, aspects that chronic pain has. It seems to have no reassuring explanation and no foreseeable end. Terminal pain has been described by Saunders (1970) as having 'no useful function, serving neither as a warning nor protection, but an illness in itself, one that has to be considered and treated as such'. Often some patients who are in a terminal stage will be so exhausted by their unrelieved condition that they will feel pain 'all over'. Attention has consequently to be paid to the whole person.

A poignant example illustrating the multiple kinds of pain in the terminal stages of cancer is quoted by Benoliel and Crowley (1973):

> I had a group of students once who took as a small study a group of patients and asked them, 'tell me about your pain'. And one old gentleman said, 'it's very interesting that you would ask, because no one ever has'. And he said, 'what kind of pain are you interested in? Are you interested in the pain that is racking my body right now and from which I will never recover? Are you asking about the pain of my life when I lost my daughter? Are you talking about the pain of my loneliness because I have no one who cares?'

It is now recognised that as many as 50 per cent of patients with advanced cancer have negligible discomfort at most or no pain at all; 40 per cent experience severe pain and the remaining 10 per cent mild to moderate pain.

Terminal pain is greatly influenced by psychological factors such as fear of disfigurement by the disease, loss of identity, the knowledge of impending death, family or financial worries, and fear of the unknown. There is also the continual dread of further pain and disease progression, coupled with the agonising uncertainty of what the future will bring. How will the family and loved ones manage? The fear of loss of dignity and control may reflect the fear of being seen in such a condition: 'I never really saw what fear was until I looked at everybody else looking at me' (Rosenthal, 1973). Family anxiety is often greatly eased when the terminally ill relative is admitted to a hospice. Thirty-four patients who died at St Christopher's Hospice were matched with thirty-four who had died in general hospitals in the area. One major difference was the amount of anxiety the spouses reported before and after admission (Hinton, 1970).

All these factors affect the sensory, affective and evaluative dimensions of terminal pain. Bond (1979) and Sternbach (1974) have shown how the cancer patient in pain develops greater anxiety, depression, hypochondriasis and neuroticism than patients with non-malignant pain. Mental pain, often harder to bear than physical pain, and therefore as important to treat, is experienced in the slow relentless destruction of the body, which in turn threatens the destruction of the social and emotional life of the individual and the family. Mental agony is far more terrible than physical pain because it can only be communicated to the few persons who are able to understand and appreciate. Fear, anxiety and depression are the most common symptoms of the mental pain of the dying. Fear is often the fear of the unknown but it may also arise from recollections of poor pain control in the past. One cancer patient described how her worst suffering was waiting for the pain that never came (Kachele, 1953). Depression can readily arise when there is the feeling of 'nothing more can be done'. Often too there are feelings of remorse and guilt which if left to themselves, unshared, become internalised and turn to resentment and bitterness. Grief becomes appropriate in those who recognise they are dying, and a sense of loss and separation can bring deep regret and pain.

Social pain is observed in the terminally ill who are afraid for the future of the spouse they are about to leave. The patient realises that the family and friends are distressed and in a sense already bereaved, and may feel guilty for having to abandon his or her children, spouse or elderly relation. Social isolation becomes very real in periods of loneliness when visitors appear less frequently or when present are rather at a loss to know how to relate, as illustrated by the following remarks by patients: 'My friends don't know what to say now that they know I know.' 'Everyone seems anxious to walk away from me.' 'The falling off of visitors hurts so much. I'm not good company now.' Involved in the social aspects of terminal pain will also be the anticipatory grief of the family, the difficulty of 'letting go'.

Feelings of helplessness, meaninglessness, failure and regret often create spiritual unrest which in turn aggravates pain. 'Why this waste?' (Matt. 26:8). As soon as Ivan in Tolstoy's novel, *The Death of Ivan Ilych*, began to sense the meaninglessness of his condition he became overwhelmed by the pain of his cancer. 'Ivan Ilych's physical sufferings were terrible, but worse than the physical sufferings were his mental sufferings, which were his chief torture.' Spiritual pain often takes the form of belief that the pain or illness has been sent as a punishment from God for past misdeeds. It is the meaningless desolation of realising that life is ending.

Terminal pain becomes a total experience with physical, mental, emotional and spiritual needs shared by both family and patient. 'Physical pains we suffer alone; mental pains, particularly grief, affect the whole circle of our acquaintances', writes Lammerton (1973), 'but the greatest pain of all, a pain of the spirit, is as great as mankind. It is the pain of a prodigal son.' One of the most common misconceptions is that dying and pain are inseparable companions, but 'one may be in pain and not be dying, or be dying and not be in pain'. Pain at death is not inevitable and although many patients still seem to experience an unnecessary amount of severe pain, in the majority of instances it is able to be relieved thanks to effective and well controlled drug therapy.

Baskerville, P. A., et al.   'Preparation for surgery: information tapes for the patient', *Practitioner*, 229 (July 1985), pp. 677–8.

Benoliel, J. Q., and Crowley, D. M.   'The patient in pain: new concepts', Proceedings of the National Conference on Cancer, *Nursing* (10 September 1973).

Berne, E. *Games that People Play: the psychology of human relationships*. Deutsch, London 1966.

Bond, M. R. *Pain: its nature, analysis and treatment.* Churchill Livingstone, Edinburgh 1979.

Bonica, J. J. 'Management of pain', *Post Graduate Medicine*, 53 (1973), pp. 56–7.
'Current status of postoperative pain therapy', in *Current Topics in Pain Research and Therapy*, ed. J. Yokota and R. Dubner (R. Excerpta Medica, Tokyo 1983), pp. 169–89.

Chapman, C. R. 'Psychological factors in postoperative pain', in G. Smith and B. G. Covino, *Acute Pain*. Butterworth, London 1985.

Engel, G. L. '"Psychogenic" pain and the pain-prone patient', *Amer. J. Med.*, 26 (1959), pp. 899–918.

Geyman, J. 'The family as the object of care in family practice', *J. Family Pract.*, 5 (1977), pp. 571–5.

Gracely, R. H. 'Psychophysical assessment of human pain', in J. J. Bonica (ed), *Advances in Pain Research and Therapy*, vol. III. Raven Press, New York 1979.

Hinton, J. 'Communication between husband and wife in terminal cancer', paper presented at Second International Conference on Social Science and Medicine, Aberdeen, 7–11 September 1970.

Jacox, A. K., and Stewart, M. 'Psychosocial contingencies of the pain experience'. Univ. Iowa College of Nursing, 1973.

Janis, I. L. *Psychological Stress*. Wiley, London 1958.

Kachele, E. *Living with Cancer*. Gollancz, London 1953.

Laing, R. D. *The Politics of Experience*. Penguin, London 1975.

Lammerton, R. 'Care of the dying: the pains of death', *Nursing Times* (11 January 1973).

Lasagna, L. 'The clinical measurement of pain', *Annals of the New York Academy of Science*, 13 (1958), pp. 28–37.

Lériche, R. *The Surgery of Pain*, tr. and ed. Archibald

41

Young. Baillière, Tindall & Cox, London 1939.

LeShan, L.
'The world of the patient in severe pain of long duration' *J. Chron. Dis.*, 17 (1964), pp. 119–26.

Loan, W. B., and Morrison, J. D.
'The incidence of severity of post-operative pain', *Brit. J. Anaesth.*, 39 (1976), pp. 695–8.

McCaffery, M.
Nursing Management of the Patient with Pain. Lippincott, Philadelphia, Pa. 1972.
Nursing the Patient in Pain, Lippincott Nursing ser. Harper & Row, London 1983.

Meinhart, N. T., and McCaffery, M.
Pain: a nursing approach to assessment and analysis. Appleton-Century-Crofts, New York 1983.

Melzack, R.
The Puzzle of Pain. Penguin, London 1978.

Melzack, R., and Torgerson, W. S.
'On the language of pain', *Anesthesiology*, 34 (1971), pp. 50–9.

Merskey, H.
'Psychological aspects of pain', *Postgrad. Med. J.*, 44 (1968), p. 297.

Rosenthal, T.
How Could I not be Among You. Avon, New York 1973.

Rowat, K. M.
'Chronic pain: a family affair', in K. King (ed.), *Long-Term Care* (Churchill Livingstone, Edinburgh 1983), pp. 137–49.

Saunders, C.
The Management of Terminal Illness. Hospital Publications, London 1967.
'The nature and management of terminal pain', in *Matters of Life and Death*, ed. E. Shotter. Darton Longman & Todd, London 1970.
Care of the Dying, Nursing Times Publication, 2nd edn, London 1976.

Sternbach, R. A.
Pain and Psychophysiological Analysis. Academic Press, New York 1968.
Pain Patients: traits and treatment. Academic Press, New York 1974.

Szaz, T. S.
Pain and Pleasure. Basic Books, New York 1957.

Twycross, R. G.
'Control of pain', *J. Roy. Coll. Physicians*, 18:1 (January 1984).

Twycross, R. G., and Lack, S. A.   *Symptom Control in Far Advanced Cancer: pain relief.* Pitman, London 1983.

Wilson-Barnett, J.   *Stress in Hospital: patients' psychological reaction to illness and health care.* Churchill Livingstone, Edinburgh 1979.

3

Relief of Pain

For the happiness mankind can gain is not in pleasure, but in rest from pain.

John Dryden (1631–1700)

Pain is soul destroying. No patient should have to endure intense pain unnecessarily. The quality of mercy is essential to the practice of medicine; here, of all places, it should not be strained.

Marcia Angell (1982)

Tolerance to pain is uniquely individual and consequently there can be no standard prescription for pain control. The experience of pain varies from person to person, from ache to agony, dependent upon the psychological reactions of the particular individual involved. To be of maximum benefit pain relief must see the patient in totality, and so take account of psychological, social and spiritual care. Teamwork is therefore essential with medical and paramedical staff, hospital chaplains and social workers, working together as members of the therapeutic team. The current methods of pain control and relief include four major approaches; pharmacological, surgical, sensory-modulatory and psychological. The primary goal of effective pain control is a pain-free patient with normal affect; to control pain so that it will not return.

DRUG THERAPY

Analgesics are the drugs of choice for the relief of most sorts of pain. Some £1,000 million is spent annually in Britain alone

44

on their purchase. Drugs which alleviate tension, anxiety and fear associated with response to pain also have a place in treatment. Their use is based on the quality and severity of the patient's pain, its cause, intensity, and probable duration.

Aspirin is the most common of all the analgesic drugs, approximately two tons being used annually. Analgesics vary in strength and can be classified as narcotic (for example, codeine and morphine) and non-narcotic (aspirin). The strong narcotics are more likely to produce side-effects. A wide range of pain-relieving agents exists. Short-acting drugs often relieve acute pain but in chronic conditions the emphasis is on preventing the recurrence of pain and so the use of longer lasting analgesics is preferable. Ideally analgesics should be given before significant pain occurs or as soon as pain begins to return. In this way severe pain can be prevented and relieved.

There is always more to analgesia than analgesics, and the importance of explaining to the patient the mechanisms underlying the pain should be emphasised. 'Pain that does not make sense or, worse, is seen as a threat, is always more intense than pain which is understandable' (Twycross, 1984). It is generally agreed that most pain, no matter how severe, can be effectively relieved by narcotic analgesics. As analgesics treat the symptoms only, it is important to evaluate fully the pathology and prognosis which might underly the disorder. Where tension, anxiety and fear are associated with the patient's response to pain, tranquillisers may be used in combination with both narcotic and non-narcotic analgesics.

PSYCHOLOGICAL PROCEDURES

Psychological procedures play an important part in pain therapy, particularly for those states which cannot be brought under satisfactory control by other methods. They are to be seen not as an alternative to drugs but rather as valuable adjuncts and are often the means of reducing prescribed dosages. A loving and caring relationship between the patient and those who minister can be an important determinant of pain relief. One patient described her feelings forty-eight hours after her operation thus:

. . . the relief of pain is not just the pills, it is the pills given with concern and caring. And if that sounds important it is. If a patient is in pain and tells a nurse, it is quite possible that, by the way the nurse moves and looks and the way she says what she says, the patient is made to feel a nuisance at least or a coward at worst. And if that happens the pain creeps up to a kind of crescendo of guilt and helplessness . . . if on the other hand there is caring – damn it, let's be honest and call it what it is – if on the other hand there is love, the pain is minimised and becomes tolerable. And mercifully, this has been the way with my pain. (Macmillan, 1980)

Another patient who was enduring terminal pain pleaded: 'Show us that we are loved – that lessens pain.' Both examples bear testimony to the importance of treating the person as well as the pain. Hinton (1972) goes as far as to state that 'if doctors and nurses set about to relieve discomfort with sincerity and competence their intention alone brings ease'.

NON-INVASIVE PAIN RELIEF

Distraction

Diversional procedures can often enhance the effects of pharmacological methods of pain relief. They are not attempts to help the patient forget about his pain but rather to provide him with alternatives. McCaffery (1979) has defined such distraction as a sensory shielding where self is protected from the pain sensation by focusing on and increasing clarity of sensations unrelated to pain. Diversion therapy is something far more fundamental than merely helping the long day to pass; it alters the amount and quality of perceived pain. It has been suggested by Saunders and Baines (1983) that 'a good gossip, like other distractions' can be one of the best ways of relieving mental pain. Listening to the radio, watching favourite TV programmes, knitting, having someone to talk to in order to release tension, are all everyday examples and help divert attention away from pain. 'I have had patients come to me', remarked a student nurse, 'and just by talking to them they have said their pain has been eased.'

Copp (1974, 1985) relates how some patients find relief in numbers and counting, and quotes the example of one patient in a burns unit, face down on a circular electric bed, who used to count tiny coloured tiles on the floor. When he reached 10,000 in one colour, he would begin to count tiles of a different colour! Other patients told of counting bricks in a wall, letters in words, flowers on draperies. Ischlondsky (1949) showed how sufferers from neuralgia and gout relieved their pain by concentrating on challenging problems. Pascal, who suffered that most painful of disorders, trigeminal neuralgia, found his helping to cope mechanism to be that of attempting to solve the problem of the cycloid (Walker, 1942). Other studies have shown that the more actively the patient participates in distraction the more effective the distraction is likely to be.

One rather bizarre form of distraction was used by a patient who was in such severe pain at home that she used to roll on the floor. The only way she could help herself was by banging her head on the floor: 'It gives me another pain to think about,' she exclaimed. Hippocrates (460–377 BC) found that 'when two pains occur together, but not in the same place, the more violent obscures the other'.

Viktor Frankl (1959), describing life in the concentration camps of the Second World War, relates how he talked to a young woman who knew she would die in the next few days yet was cheerful in spite of this knowledge. Pointing through the window of her camp hut, she said, 'This tree here is the only friend I have in my loneliness.' Through that window she could see just one branch of a chestnut tree, and on the branch were two blossoms. 'I often talk to this tree,' she told Frankl. Anxiously he asked her if the tree replied. On being told 'yes, it did' he then asked her, 'What did it say?' She answered, 'It said to me, "I am here – I am here – I am life, eternal life".' Under similar conditions in wartime concentration camps Corrie ten Boom (1971) in her suffering and mental torture was able to thank God for the distraction of fleas!

Occupational and physiotherapy

Occupational therapists are integral members of the treatment programme for patients with chronic pain. They help sufferers to assume control and responsibility for their lives by developing various skills in the areas of work, play and self-care. Arts and crafts activities can reassure a patient of his ability to function on some level. Occupational therapy can also serve as a distraction and involve the patient's active participation, which in itself has therapeutic effect. The more the chronically ill patient can do for himself and the more interests he can develop the better the quality of his life. In this way the occupational therapist helps the patient become less pain-orientated and more activity-orientated. The goal of treatment is not 'cure' but rather the achievement of the maximum level of psychosocial functioning possible for the patient concerned.

Physiotherapists will also function as important members of the relief team, for massage, relaxation and breathing exercises all help to release tension and so alleviate the pain experience.

Music

Since the days of David and Saul music and medicine have been closely associated. 'When the evil spirit from God was upon Saul . . . David took an harp, and played with his hand: so Saul was refreshed, and was well, and the evil spirit departed from him' (1 Sam. 16:23). 'Art thou troubled, music will calm thee': throughout the centuries physicians, priests, musicians and philosophers have all acknowledged the tranquillising and healing effect of music. 'Who hears music', wrote Browning (1871), 'feels his solitude peopled at once.'

Locsin (1981) studied the effect of music on the pain of a selected group of postoperative patients during the first forty-eight hours after surgery, and showed that attention can be distracted by refocusing it to a pleasant sensory stimulus, particularly music, which works as a distraction medium. Music occupied the patients' minds with something familiar, soothing and preferred. When these patients were asked how music affected their postoperative pain 88 per cent answered that it 'lessened the pain', while 33 per cent replied that music 'distracted' them from the pain. It was found that those who listened to music needed less pain-relief medication. Rhythmic movement can serve as a distraction and the patient might be encouraged to keep time by tapping his feet or fingers. It should be explained to him that distraction is a short-term pain relief measure, and care should be taken to prevent him becoming bored or overtired.

One patient said that a friend had suggested a musical aid:

> On one side of a tape I recorded loud, fast, rock music, which I played when I was in pain. One can absorb just so many stimuli, and when I concentrated on the music, the painful stimulus was not so strong. The other side, a recording of soft, slow, gentle music helped me relax when I was not experiencing pain. (Cady, 1976)

Music therapy in the palliative care of patients with advanced malignant disease was observed by Munro and Mount (1978). They found a broad variety of uses of music. *Physically* it assisted in muscular relaxation and broke the vicious circle of chronic pain by relieving anxiety and depression, thus altering the perception of pain. *Psychologically* it provided a non-verbal means of expressing a broad range of recognised and unconscious feelings. *Socially* it served as a bond and sense of community with family members and others, as a link to the patient's life before the illness, and as entertainment and diversion. *Spiritually* it provided means of expressing spiritual feelings, and provided an avenue for expressing doubts, anger, and questions on the ultimate meaning of life.

Over the past few decades there has been a fluctuation of interest in musical programming during dental procedures as a method of obtaining patient relaxation and even a degree of analgesia during treatment. For a number of patients audio-analgesia was so effective that no other analgesic or anaes-thetic agent was needed. Dentists have long recognised that relaxation appears to actually reduce distress or anxiety, whereas distraction helps the patient temporarily to ignore the distress. Many patients comment on the extent to which their engrossment in music diverts them from attending to details of the treatment procedures.

Selections of music when used need to be carefully chosen, and patient preferences seem to be a key factor. Ischlondsky

(1949) found that a Bach fugue raised the pain threshold 26 per cent for a classical musician but a popular tune raised the threshold only 8 per cent. A young college student experienced the reverse.

Relaxation

Relaxation reduces tension and thereby minimises pain. In the early 1930s Grantley Dick-Read greatly decreased the pains of childbirth by teaching conscious relaxation in labour. Not only does relaxation accompanied by rhythmic breathing diminish pain but also greatly assists patients to rest and sleep better. It is impossible to relax and at the same time worry or be anxious. A patient in postoperative pain related that 'relaxation techniques were of enormous value. When the pain was particularly severe, nurses coached me to relax individual muscles, beginning with my forehead. This not only relaxed the muscles, a source of back pain, but it diverted my attention from the pain.' In such a calm state of mind we are better able to cope with pain.

Relaxation exercises are most effective if they can be learned when the intensity of pain is at its lowest. Methods of relaxation are particularly helpful for patients who suffer from headaches, migraine and disorders where muscle tension plays a part. A study undertaken by Wilson (1981) with patients hospitalised for elective surgery and randomly assigned into four categories: (a) control; (b) information; (c) relaxation training; and (d) relaxation training with information; found that the latter group reported the greatest reduction of pain and pain medication. Yoga exercises also achieve an extremely high level of muscular relaxation. Pain produces muscle spasm and whatever method helps systematically to relax muscles becomes a therapeutic tool.

Physical touch

The use of touch to relieve discomfort and to heal has been acknowledged throughout the history of mankind yet it is a somewhat neglected field – 'the lost dimension of the physical'. According to Desmond Morris (1971), 'we often talk about the way we talk, and we frequently try to see the way we see, but for some reason we have rarely touched on the way we touch'! Physical touch connects us with our humanness. In the New Testament many of the healing works of Jesus were performed through the laying on of hands. In the apostolic church the disciples reflected the theme that 'salvation' included physical, mental and spiritual health. In Mark 16:18 the disciples are told that they 'shall lay hands on the sick, and they shall recover'.

Touch is a medium through which persons repeatedly communicate and it is only through communication that man's greatest need as a human being, the need to love and be loved, is fulfilled. Physical touch is also a symbol of identification. A most vivid example is that of Thomas who doubted that Jesus had risen from the dead and was not convinced until he had touched the living Christ: 'Then saith he to Thomas, reach hither thy finger, and behold my hands; and reach thither thy hand, and thrust it into my side: and be not faithless, but believing. And Thomas answered and said unto him, My Lord and my God' (John 20:27–8). Touch can express feelings and reactions, which in turn can be conveyed to others.

Holding hands, putting an arm round the patient, are expressions of affection and friendliness. Kubler-Ross (1969) found that the most expressive relationship during terminal illness was a gentle pressure of the hand in moments of silence. Physical actions symbolise that someone understands, encourages and comforts. Anna Freud (1952) has described how the youngest blitz victims of the Second World War maintained their morale in the midst of rubble and wreckage when they had a living and helping hand to cling to. The simple holding of a hand can be the outward and tangible sign of inward acceptance. In that act we are saying what cannot be said adequately in words. Love – agape – becomes elevated as a mark of genuine community, not so much an idea floating around in thought and words but the sharing of person with person. For a patient in pain touch helps to locate him in time and space; he is not alone, someone is present who has time to listen and to comfort. 'I am here to be with you.' Feelings of relaxation and peace often follow as a consequence. 'I am much more calm and peaceful now.'

Imagery

People learn to cope with pain by adopting various methods and techniques. It has already been noted how distraction and relaxation help the mind of many a patient to become diverted from the painful event. Imagery is a procedure employed to conjure up the most vivid possible picture or scene which is incompatible with pain. It may include one or all the senses of vision, hearing, movement, touch, smell and taste. The patient is encouraged to visualise an idyllic pastoral scene and imagine himself far away from his present predicament. He can also be asked to describe his favourite place, holiday or pleasurable experience; people known, places visited, routes travelled can all be recalled.

Mental visualisation can include deep concentration exercises such as reorganising cupboards and drawers, going through the attic, cleaning up the desk, sewing specific stitches in imaginery needlework. Imagery helps to promote relaxation and this in turn alleviates or eliminates the anxiety accompanying physical discomfort and decreases pain. Mental imagining creates a milieu which stimulates the patient's own natural healing processes. The ultimate aim of this method is to decrease the intensity of pain, and in some instances it may eliminate it completely. Much of its effectiveness however depends upon the image used and the ability of the patient concerned.

Meditation

Meditation involves achievement of deep relaxation and the concentration of the attention on a single thought or theme. This is accompanied by a peace of mind and sense of well-being which neutralise strain and stress. One method which may be so used is transcendental meditation (TM) where the person relaxes in a passive attitude with eyes closed. A 'mantra', a pre-selected word, sound or phrase, signifying 'rest', 'peace', 'healing', 'wholeness', is the source of meditation for about 15 to 20 minutes twice daily. TM exercises have been used specifically to release neuro-muscular tensions in local areas of the body. Studies (Benson, 1974; Lindermann, 1973; and Rathbone, 1969) have observed that patients who practised methods of meditation or yoga had very low blood pressure during periods of meditation. Relaxation of the mind in meditation helps to break the vicious circle of stress-pain-stress-anxiety. The mind is calmed by the repetition and soothing sounds or phrases, and thus the patient gains self-control in relation to his responses to pain.

Copp (1974) found that many patients seem to concentrate on various words, of which there are eight major sorts:

control: 'I won't scream'; 'I can stand this';
supplication: 'Hear me'; 'Let it be over soon';
intercession: 'Help me, Jesus';
memorised words: prayers, psalms, mnemonic devices;
repetitive: nonsensical, short-staccato and many-syllabled words;
derisive: 'This is stupid';
evaluative: 'It hurts most now'; 'It's coming again'; 'It's going to ease off soon';
anxious: 'I can't make it through this'.

In a study of religion in patients with advanced cancer Yates et al. (1981) found that belief in a power greater than man and the helpfulness of prayer and meditation showed particularly strong negative correlation with pain level. They conclude that there is considerable evidence that people's reports of pain are greatly influenced by their attitude towards it, and it is possible that religious views and connections are associated with an attitude that results in a lessened experience of pain. The common element seems to be 'getting outside of oneself'. In another study of cancer patients by Mount (1984) emphasis is placed on the importance of personal transcendence when 'material things and events may be recognised as ultimately of limited value', and 'the significance of time, feelings, and relationships may be seen in a new perspective'. When this is so the significance of the patient's cancer pain may be transformed, 'for it is when we are down and experiencing a time of adversity that we may be most willing to open the doors of our personality and expose our needs'.

Meditation might also take the form of the recalling of passages from Scripture with affirmations and ejaculatory prayers repeated slowly and thoughfully. Such deep meditation, when it becomes practical in painful circumstances, enables a person to attain inner peace and concentration and expel extraneous environmental distractions. Pain then gets offered up to God.

> Try more and more at the moment [of pain] itself, without any delay or evasion, without any fixed form, as simply and spontaneously as possible, to cry out to God, to Christ our Lord, in any way that comes most handy, and the more variously the better . . . the all important point is, to make them [ejaculations] at the time and with the pain well mixed up into the prayer. (von Hugel, 1964)

Those who are able to feel close to God often find that their religious faith and experience help to lessen their pain or at least make it more bearable.

Hypnotherapy

Hypnosis is a state of mind in which the subject shows increased susceptibility to suggestions made by the therapist. Quiet, warmth, comfort and a relaxing atmosphere will aid successful induction of hypnosis. Concentration is centred around a pleasing, calm and peaceful scene in which the patient is encouraged to participate. In this way anxiety, fear, pain and stress can be alleviated. Some studies have shown that 15 to 20 per cent of hypnotisable patients with moderate to severe pain can achieve total relief with hypnosis. By lowering the burden of emotional suffering, pain may become bearable. Some awareness of the pain has to be retained because of its protective function as a warning system. A few patients have been able to be hypnotised sufficiently deeply to undergo major surgery without anaesthesia. However hypnosis does not appear to be effective for any form of chronic pain, and Melzack and Wall (1982) doubt whether hypnotic suggestion is any better than a placebo pill and encouragement or moral support from the family physician and parish priest.

Placebo

Researchers have demonstrated that about a third of patients receive significant pain relief through the use of placebos. The word 'placebo' is derived from the Latin verb meaning 'I shall please'. (It appears as the first word in the ninth verse of Psalm 114 in the Vulgate.) The placebo effect has been thought to be due to suggestion, distraction, the patient's optimism that something is being done, or the desire to please the doctor. There is much evidence to suggest that placebos are as potent as drugs. Cousins and Schiefelbein (1978) suggest that the placebo is powerful not because it 'fools the body', but because it translates the will to live into a physical reality by triggering specific biochemical changes in the body. It appears that it is the respect for the source of a placebo which is the important factor in its effectiveness.

A placebo has been defined by McCaffery (1979) as 'any medical treatment that produces an effect in a patient because of its implicit or explicit therapeutic intent, and not because of its specific nature'. It should not be implied that because people are helped by placebos they do not suffer real pain, for no one denies the reality of either acute or chronic pain. Melzack and Wall (1982) reveal that placebos are more effective for severe pain than for mild pain, and are more effective when patients are under great stress and anxiety than when they are not. They also make the interesting comment that two placebo capsules seem to be more effective than one, and large capsules better than small ones! It is evident that a placebo becomes more potent when accompanied by the strong suggestion that a powerful analgesic has been given. They conclude that the greater the implicit and explicit suggestion that pain will be relieved the greater the relief obtained by the patient.

In a study by Lasagna et al. (1954) of the placebo effect on postoperative patients, it was found that when patients suffering from steady, severe wound pain were injected subcutaneously with 1 ml saline, three or four out of every ten reported satisfactory relief of pain. What remains unanswered is why some patients respond positively to placebos while others do not, and why some patients respond consistently while others respond only occasionally. Patients who are able to obtain pain relief from placebos are classified as 'placebo reactors', while those who do not gain benefit are 'non reactors'. It is interesting to compare the personalities of the placebo reactors with those of the nonreactors. There appear to be significant differences in attitudes, habits, educational backgrounds, and personality structures.

PHYSICAL THERAPY

Acupuncture

Acupuncture is a traditional form of Chinese medicine which has been in practice for at least two thousand years. It is the technique of inserting fine needles under the skin at selected points in the body, the acupuncture points which lie upon specific lines known as 'meridians'. The Chinese recognise the existence of a Master Energy known as 'chi' in the human body, and this 'chi' energy supposedly circulates in twelve channels (meridians). The oriental explanation for the effectiveness of acupuncture in the relief of pain is the concept that disharmony between the universal life forces called 'yin' and 'yang' causes pain and diseases. When the acupuncture needles are inserted at specific points the two opposites (yin and yang) regain harmony.

Acupuncture has become known in the West only since the early 1970s and there are now an increasing number of practitioners at work in this country. Accurate assessments of its efficacy are extremely difficult to establish but some studies show an initial reduction in pain in roughly 60 per cent of cases treated. Those patients who are most likely to be helped suffer from headaches, migraines, and musculoskeletal disorders. Anxiety is often allayed when the patient's faith in the procedure is encouraged and the acupuncturist's suggestions accepted. There are continuing studies being carried out to search for a physiological basis for its effectiveness as a method of pain relief. Current opinion is that more controlled trials are needed to define which pain conditions might be helped by acupuncture and which patients are most likely to benefit. At present only a small percentage of patients seem to respond to acupuncture treatment.

Transcutaneous electric nerve stimulator

A transcutaneous electric nerve stimulator (TENS) is a battery-powered device that when switched on transmits an electrical impulse to the body through electrodes attached to the skin. The stimulation yields much pain relief in some chronic pain patients. It works best when applied to the skin near where the pain is felt and where other sensibilities like touch or pressure have not been damaged. Several kinds of TENS are available and their success rate varies greatly. It is estimated that the majority of chronic pain patients obtain from 75 to 85 per cent relief: but some patients get no relief, while others seem to have total relief. A person who has suffered intractable pain for a long time welcomes any amount of relief. In order to obtain the best results patients usually need to use the machine, which can be worn undetected under clothing, for several hours a day. It has major advantages over narcotic analgesics as it has no side-effects; it does not create respiratory depression or decreased consciousness levels. TENS has not proved to be helpful in cancer pain requiring narcotic analgesics. It can be used in such patients to help control residual pain due more to muscle tension – pain due to benign lesions rather than malignant ones.

Recent trials are being carried out to confirm the usefulness of TENS in reducing labour pain in childbirth. Medical progress has not yet resolved the difficult problem of removing the pain of labour contractions without harming the mother or the baby. It is hoped that the use of TENS will increase the production of endorphine, which is the body's own natural analgesia, during the relaxation phase of the uterus. A continuous current is released during contractions to prevent impulses reaching the brain.

Surgical procedures

In certain circumstances surgical procedures are used to alleviate pain. Surgery is not normally a first line of treatment, but is used in those instances where all other conventional measures have continually proved of no avail. The majority of surgical procedures are directed towards the interruption or destruction of sensory pathways to the cerebrum. There are a variety of operations to relieve pain, the most common being cordotomy, which is the severing of the nerve fibres on one or both sides of the spinal cord that travel the express routes to the brain. Surgery within the brain or the spinal cord to relieve pain includes severing connections at the major junctions in pain pathways. Sometimes surgeons can relieve pain by destroying nerve fibres outside the brain or spinal cord, such as the destruction of sympathetic nerves. Nerve blocks, which damage or cut the nerve endings, are often spectacularly successful in controlling pain situations in both operative and postoperative stages. They are usually successful in the symptoms of chronic states such as cancer pain. Nerve blocks however are rarely permanent and may have to be repeated in a matter of months. The long-term success rates of surgical intervention are rather disappointing. It is estimated that pain returns to the majority of patients at any period from six to eighteen months after surgery (Sternbach, 1978).

Although the above therapies, non-invasive pain relief methods, and physical therapies may not abolish pain completely at least they make it more bearable for variable periods of time.

THE GENERAL PRACTITIONER

'How many adult human beings are there, now, at this minute, rushing about in mute panic wishing they could find a doctor', says the old physician in *Cancer Ward* (Solzhenitsyn, 1968), 'the kind of person to whom they can pour out the fears they have deeply concealed.'

It is often the general practitioner who has the initial contact with those in pain, and it is estimated that two out of every three patients who consult their family doctor have problems of pain. The majority of these expect the doctor to have the answer to all their various ills, and consequently the relief of pain is probably the most frequent demand made upon the physician.

One of the most common of all pains is that classified as 'headache'. Normally some 90 per cent of the population suffer from this discomfort at one time or another. Headaches seem to occur in women more than men and most frequently in the age-span between puberty and the climacteric. Tension headache, involving continual contractions of head and neck muscles, is one of the most common forms. Another variety is the vascular headache such as migraine which is associated with throbbing pain on one side of the head.

Apart from headaches, low back pain is the most painful complaint encountered in general practice. At least one out of every two people in western society suffers from back trouble at some time in his life. A study undertaken by Ingham and Miller (1979) reported that 21 per cent of a random selected sample of people aged between sixteen and seventy-five, who had not visited their general practitioner for at least three months, declared themselves to be suffering from back pain when interviewed.

More than two million people a year in the United Kingdom consult their family doctors because of back pain alone. The DHSS Working Group on Back Pain (1979) estimated that 11.5 million days are lost annually on account of this trouble. Backache thus causes more time off work than strikes. Stubbs et al. (1981) state that an estimated 185,000 nurses (43 per cent of the NHS total nursing population of England and Wales) will suffer back pain at least once a year. Approximately 1.1 million patients consult their GP: of these 0.3 million are referred to hospital; 30,000 are admitted to hospital; and 5,000 have an operation on their back (Waddell, 1982). The total annual cost of backache in the United Kingdom is nearly £1,000 million.

Arthritic conditions also are among the most painful attended by general practitioners. Arthritis, which is one of the most crippling disorders, accounts for the loss of 85 million working days in Britain each year. The worst affected areas appear to be the north-west of England and Wales, losing more than 9 million working days at a cost of more than £285 million. According to a Report (1986) of the Arthritis and Rheumatism Council (ARC) 3.31 working days per year are lost for every member of the population in Wales, compared to 0.97 days in the south of England. This high figure is probably due to the large number of people working in heavy industries, who are more likely to develop the complaint.

The most common forms of the disease are osteoarthritis and rheumatoid arthritis. Fortunately there is now more hope of pain relief for people with rheumatic diseases, thanks to research being undertaken by ARC. It is now known that over a third of people with rheumatoid arthritis recover completely. Through further advances in genetic engineering it is hoped that a preventive drug to protect people from arthritis may become available, perhaps within the next five to ten years.

More than 25 per cent of patients visiting their general practitioners have emotional, psychological or psychiatric problems. Gomez and Dally (1977) found that no less than 84 per cent of patients with abdominal pain in medical and surgical clinics were there for psychological reasons. 'They complain of physical pain,' commented one family doctor, 'but their real problem is emotional – a marital problem, a broken relationship. It is extremely difficult to get them to accept that emotional problems might well be the cause of their pain.' Many patients are frightened and this makes their pain threshold much lower. Another GP said:

> People who have pure physical pain are usually very descriptive. They will say, 'I have a sharp pain in my chest'. These are a comparatively easy group with which to deal. People who say, 'I have a headache which is like a tight band around my head', 'a pain in my chest which is like flames', or 'It's just something I feel inside me', usually have a strong emotional element as well. The natural reaction is to give them something or do something for them to relieve their pain. That is a very natural attitude and it's difficult sometimes to stand by, but you first have to diagnose and then treat.

The task of the general practitioner is far more family-orientated than that of the hospital physician and the pain experiences of his patients may expose family tensions. 'I often find this more emotionally draining than the physical condition of my patients,' confessed an experienced practitioner, 'we live with our patients throughout most of their lives.' Pain is heightened as a result of broken interpersonal relationships. Many a family makes great sacrifices, particularly in cases of chronic or terminal illness at home. 'There was amazing strength and courage where I originally perceived weakness', was a typical comment of a number of doctors who were reflecting on the family environment.

'Lots of people basically want reassurance, and not necessarily treatment,' stated a recently qualified doctor in a large group practice. 'They want to know what the pain is. Many a patient on being told, for example, "You've strained your back", will reply, "Fine, I can put up with the pain now that I know what it is. I don't need any pain-killers".' Surveys conducted on the expectations and experience of patients who consult in a training practice seem to bear this out. Bradley (1981) observed that of all the patients (348) seen in one week in a training practice in Exeter, 'to be told what was wrong' was the single commonest expectation (92 per cent). Just over half expected a prescription, 38 per cent sought advice or help and a further 23 per cent sought suggestions for self-help. These people seem to be requesting the 'drug doctor' (Balint, 1957) at least as strongly as conventional drugs. All the questions dealing with verbal communication between doctor and patient produced uniformly high expectation rates, much higher than those dealing with doctor actions. These people did not share the medical urge 'to do something'. Consistent findings of previous studies have been that more people receive a prescription than expect one.

THE HOSPICE

There are many patients who do not need the highly techno-logical approach of the large hospital yet cannot be cared for at home. For such as these the ideal setting is the small specialised environment of the hospice or continuing care unit. The prime purpose of hospice care was graphically defined by one terminally ill patient: 'I am a traveller on the journey from one life to the next, and I need a place where I can be welcomed and looked after and cared for and be myself on that journey' (Hadlock, 1983).

In 1985 there was a total of 101 in-patient hospice units throughout Britain, consisting of fifty-four independent free-standing hospices run by registered charities; thirteen Macmillan Continuing Care homes built in NHS grounds, with the revenue costs paid by the NHS and the capital costs paid by the charity Cancer Relief; eight other Macmillan 'mini-units', funded in a similar manner to the Continuing Care homes; six Sue Ryder homes; eleven Marie Curie Foundation homes; and finally nine Continuing Care wards in

NHS hospitals funded by the NHS. The distribution of hospice units throughout the country is somewhat uneven. East Anglia, Wales and the north are poorly serviced, while there is a more adequate provision in the south (particularly the London area), the west Midlands and the south-west.

Studies have found that people dying at home and in hospital may suffer much unnecessary pain. On the other hand it has been shown that severe pain can nearly always be controlled in hospices and similar special units. Parkes (1978) observed that people dying at home although much more likely to remain mobile and in clear consciousness than those dying in hospital, were also more likely to suffer more pain. One of the unfortunate reasons appeared to be that of inadequate pain relief. This might have been due partly to the failure of the patient's general practitioner to ensure that regular doses of the appropriate analgesics were given in sufficient dosage to prevent the pain from becoming severe, or to arrange for admission to hospital if this failed. There often appears to be an inadequate concept of pain, coupled with the fear (ill grounded) concerning the addictive effects of narcotic analgesics. Other factors reflected misunderstandings on the part of the patient or members of his family.

A study by Hunt et al. (1977) revealed that much pain seems to go unrecognised in a general teaching hospital, where 'nurses accept the presence of unrelieved pain in patients too readily, as indicated by the practice of confining enquiry about pain to drug rounds and by ignoring non-verbal communications'. Greater importance seems to be given to the use of analgesics than to other methods of elevating the pain threshold. One patient entering a hospice, having been discharged from a general hospital, remarked: 'It was so strange no one seemed to want to look at me.' In a later study Parkes (1980) observed that over 20 per cent of patients at home with terminal cancer had unsatisfactory relief from pain. The findings of Parkes' research are not dissimiliar from those of Cartwright (1973) who reported pain present in 66 per cent of a stratified sample of 785 patients who had died (from all causes). Parkes reports the extent to which pain was relieved in three groups of patients:

(a) of hospital-centred patients 20 per cent suffered severe and mostly unrelieved pain;
(b) home centred patients became an increasing problem, 6 per cent experienced unrelieved pain prior to the final period and rose to 28 per cent during the final phase of care at home;
(c) patients admitted to St Christopher's Hospice showed a reduction in severe and unrelieved pain from 36 per cent in the pre-terminal period to 8 per cent in the terminal phase.

When patients are admitted to hospices or special-care relief units there is normally a striking improvement in their pain symptoms.

The hospice movement and its teaching stands for far more than procedures and techniques of pain-control. It not only addresses the full spectrum of the needs of the patient in pain but also offers practical application to the essential values of life. It also relies heavily on the total caring attitudes of its staff. The patient is allowed to remain a 'person' and is not seen as another 'case' but as an integrated personality with not only physical dimensions but also intellectual, emotional, social and spiritual needs. He is helped to be himself rather than be forced to put on a bold front or a protective façade; he is helped to realise that death is not an ending but a beginning, not a departing but an arriving, not a defeat but a victory. Family and patient are seen together as a unit of care.

The areas in which these units differ from the other existing traditional services have been outlined by Mount (1984). They assign a high priority to psychosocial and spiritual issues in addition to their basic concern – excellence in physical care. The patient and the family, not the patient alone, constitute the unit of care. An attempt is made to focus on personality and to counter institutional dehumanisation. A hospice staff nurse who had previously worked on the wards of a large district general hospital described some of the distinguishing features of hospice care:

One of the chief differences between the hospice and the general hospital is the concept of care. We are trying to create a different type of environment. We have to face up to the fact that the majority of our patients we are not going to be able to cure. At some stage they are going to die. In the general hospital ward the staff would aim to diagnose, treat and hopefully send the patient home cured. We are here to provide skilled and caring services to those for whom cure may no longer be a feasible option . . . we see ourselves as a symptom-control unit but we do not stop there, for pain is not solely a physical problem. We also look at the psychosocial and spiritual aspects of total care. If you create the right type of environment all other things seem to fall into place.

In the 'therapeutic milieu' of the hospice members of the family are encouraged to participate in patient care: time is taken to listen to the family and to understand their concerns. Family meetings are arranged in order to assist in communication and the expression of feelings. Against such a background interpersonal tensions are more readily alleviated and resolved, and in turn contribute to pain relief.

In a 'spiritual continuum' of intense caring and compassion, patients are helped to see themselves as whole persons, to gain reassurance and hope, so that they are able to live the remainder of their lives free from pain and other distressing symptoms, and so maximise the present quality of living for as long as life itself lasts. They are able to witness other patients around them who have their pain controlled and remain mentally alert. All this helps to resolve many of their own personal fears and fantasies. Some of the basic principles of the hospice environment are described by Walsh and Saunders (1984):

There must be readiness for the cost of commitment and a continual search for meaning. Devotion has been an outstanding characteristic of past and present hospices . . . affirmation of faith may be made but never imposed: each individual has to grow into a fuller (though never complete) realisation of the truths he accepts. In such a climate patients and families are encouraged to reach out towards what they see as true.

Included in the concept is also that of 'staff pain', to work through the strains and stresses of the whole supportive team. Provision must be made for the care of the hospice team to enable them to cope successfully with feelings of stress. In a BBC interview Saunders (1983) described the strain: 'Hospice work is very taxing . . . we in this work are always somehow missing an outer layer of skin and we must take care to renew ourselves.'

The aim of hospice care is to anticipate and prevent pain rather than treat it. Appropriate amounts of analgesics are administered regularly without waiting for the pain to reappear. Drugs are given at fixed intervals rather than being dispensed at a p.r.n. regimen (an abbreviation of the Latin *pro re nata*, 'according to circumstances' or 'when required or needed'). Frequently under normal conditions p.r.n. narcotic is administered when pain is present. One of the major principles laid down by Twycross (1972) in dealing with terminal pain is: 'Thou shalt not use the abbreviation p.r.n.' There is a careful balance observed between the needs of the individual and the drugs and dosages used. Pain is relieved by giving regular small doses of analgesics even if there is no pain at the time the drug is given. As far as possible pain is not allowed to return and the memory and fear of it are broken.

The primary aim of effective pain control is a pain-free patient with normal affect, that is, the patient can sustain a mentally alert state without any of the drug-induced drowsiness or euphoria which is so often an unfortunate reaction under other conditions. It allows him to maintain some degree of control over the final stages of his life, and relieves him of becoming dependent upon the ward drug round and the ward clock. He is helped to participate in decisions, and to make what time remains to him satisfying and serene without the threat and fear of pain. For a large number of patients it is now possible for their pain problems to be effectively alleviated.

Many of the hospices have a service working in collaboration with the general practitioner and primary care team. The concept of hospice care has also been extended into some general hospitals by symptom control teams, which are multidisciplinary and advise the medical and nursing staff in the wards of the hospitals concerned. In the hospices numbers of volunteers are enlisted to work together with the professional staff, so involving the whole community in a loving and caring concern.

PAIN CLINICS

The establishment of pain clinics in hospitals is increasing in all areas of the United Kingdom. They offer facilities for the specialised treatment of those patients with intractable chronic pain. There are a number of units, such as the clinic at the Royal Marsden Hospital, London, which specialise in certain sorts of pain. Their central aim is not so much the management of pain as the treatment of it, and they represent the ideal in pain-care and relief. The normal pattern in the United Kingdom is for the clinic to be set within the hospital with all the necessary facilities at hand, access to day-beds (or where needed in-patient beds), and the support team of medical, paramedical and nursing staff. A consultant anaesthetist is normally in charge who refers to colleagues in other specialties whenever the need arises. (Anaesthetists manage some 98 per cent of British pain clinics.) Social workers, physiotherapists and occupational therapists also provide supportive therapy. Patients are normally referred by local general practitioners and hospital consultants. The staff-patient relationship plays a vital role in the treatment programme, as a member of staff at a pain clinic explained:

> When people come in here they are made to feel a *person*, not just a patient . . . The caring attitude of the nurses is very important – they need to understand that the patient's pain is real – it is very important to assess the whole patient, particularly in relation to his anxiety level . . .

The majority of patients attending pain clinics suffer from intractable pain, that is, pain whose cause cannot be discovered and which has proved resistant to conventional treatment. The variety of patients treated would include those suffering from malignant disease, neuralgia, low back pain, rheumatoid arthritis, osteoarthritis, neck pain. One of the advantages of treatment at a pain clinic is improvement of function for the patient, for many have suffered chronic pain and immobility over a long period of time. The staff provide all modern methods of treatment, invasive and non-invasive, physical, psychological and pharmacological.

A pain clinic has four major functions – diagnostic, therapeutic, teaching and research. One doctor who works in a pain relief centre relates how:

> many of the patients who arrive at the clinic have a feeling they have been 'discarded' that 'nothing more can be done'. We do not relieve all the patients by any means. Pain is a crutch on which to lean; it is a cry for help and the cry needs interpreting – sometimes the need is not for medicine, sometimes the cause is socio-economic. We help many and we prevent others from succumbing to escalating drugs or neuro-surgical operations – and there is every hope that we will do better still. (Swerdlow 1978)

About half the patients in a pain relief clinic receive some form of nerve block as definitive treatment. Co-operation with the patient's general practitioner is of the utmost importance. The earlier the treatment is carried out the better the results are likely to be, so early referral is vital. An understanding of the patient's family and home circumstances are also highly desirable.

Those in pain need all the support and care that it is possible to give them to alleviate their condition. The lives of many in chronic pain, particularly those who live alone or have little emotional rapport with their families, often appear meaningless and despairing. Our prime duty is to be aware of their needs. It was Hinton (1972) who, addressing members of the medical profession, stated: 'We emerge deserving of little credit; we who are capable of ignoring the conditions which make muted people suffer. The dissatisfied dead cannot noise abroad the negligence they have suffered.' Such an indictment becomes equally applicable to all members of modern society.

ARC Report   *Arthritis in Industry*, Report of Arth. & Rheum. Council (January 1986).

Balint, M.   *The Doctor, his Patient and the Illness.* Pitman, London 1957.

Benson, H., et al.   'The Relaxation Response' *Psychiatry*, 37
                        (1974), pp. 37, 46.
                        The Relaxation Response. Avon Books, New
                        York, 1976
Boom, C. ten   *The Hiding Place.* Hodder & Stoughton,
                        London 1971.
Bradley, N. C. A.   'Expectations and experience of people who
                        consult a training practice', *J. Roy. Coll.
                        Gen. Pract.*, 31 (1981), pp. 420–5.
Browning, R.   Balaustion's Adventure, 1871.
Cady, J. W.   'Dear Pain', *Am. J. Nursing*, 76:6 (1976),
                        pp. 950–1.
Cartwright, A.   *Human Relations and Hospital Care.* Free Press
                        of Glencoe, London 1963.
                        Life Before Death. Routledge & Kegan Paul,
                        London 1973.
Copp, L. A.   'The spectrum of suffering', *Am. J. Nursing*,
                        74:3 (1974), pp. 491–5.
                        (ed.) *Recent Advances in Nursing: Perspectives
                        on Pain.* Churchill Livingstone, Edinburgh
                        1985.
Cousins, N., and   'Medicine's miracle cure: the placebo,'
   Schiefelbein, S.   *Reader's Digest* (1978), pp. 67–9.
DHSS   *Report of Working Group on Back Pain*, Dept
                        Health & Soc. Sec. HMSO, London
                        1979.
Dick-Read, G.   *Natural Childbirth.* Heinemann, London
                        1933.
Frankl, V.   *From Death-Camp to Existentialism.* Beacon
                        Press, Boston, USA 1959.
Freud, A.   'The role of bodily illness in the mental life
                        of children', in *The Psychoanalytical Study of
                        the Child*, VII (1952).
Gomez, J., and   'Psychologically mediated abdominal pain
   Dally, P.   in surgical and medical outpatient clinics',
                        Brit. Med. J. 1 (6074) (1977), pp. 1451–3.
Hinton, J.   *Dying*, 2nd edn. Penguin, London 1972.
                        'Comparison of places and policies for
                        terminal care', *Lancet*, 1 (8106) (1979),
                        pp. 29–32.
Hugel, B. von   *Spiritual Counsels and Letters*, ed. D. V. Steere.
                        Darton, Longman & Todd, London 1964.

Hunt, J., et al.	'Patients with protracted pain: a survey conducted at the London Hospital', *J. Med. Eth.*, 4:2 (1977).
Ingham, J. G., and Miller, P. McC.	'Symptom prevalence and severity in general practice population', *Brit. J. Prev. Soc. Med.*, 33:3. (September 1979), pp. 191–8.
Ischlondsky, N. E.	*Brain and Behavior.* St Louis, Mosby 1949.
Kubler-Ross, E.	*On Death and Dying.* Macmillan, New York 1969.
Lasagna, L., et al.	'A study of the placebo response', *Amer. J. Med.* (June 1954), pp. 770–9.
Lindermann, H.	*Relieve Tension the Autogenic Way.* Wyden, New York 1973.
Locsin, R. G. R. A. C.	'The effect of music on the pain of selected post-operative patients', *J. Adv. N.*, 6 (1981), pp. 19–25.
Macmillan, P.	'Thinking aloud', *Nursing Times* (6 March 1980), p. 403.
McCaffery, M.	*Nursing Management of the Patient with Pain.* Lippincott, New York 1979.
Melzack, R., and Wall, P. D.	*The Challenge of Pain.* Penguin, London 1982.
Morris, D.	*Intimate Behaviour.* Book Club Associates, London 1971.
Mount, B. M.	'Psychological and social aspects of cancer pain', in *Textbook of Pain*, ed. P. D. Wall and R. Melzack. Churchill Livingstone, Edinburgh 1984.
Munro, S., and Mount, B. M.	'Music therapy in palliative care', *Canadian Med. Assoc. J.*, 119 (1978), pp. 1029–34.
Parkes, C. M.	'Home or hospital? Terminal care as seen by surviving spouses', *J. Roy. Coll. Gen. Pract.*, 28 (186) (1978), pp. 19–30. 'Terminal care: evaluation of an advisory domiciliary service at St Christopher's Hospice', *Post. Med. J.*, 56 (660) (1980), pp. 685–9.
Rathbone, J.	*Relaxation.* Lea & Febiger, Philadelphia 1969.
Saunders, C. M., and Baines, M.	*Living with Dying: the management of terminal disease.* OUP 1983.
Solzenitsyn, A. J.	*Cancer Ward.* Penguin, London 1968.

Sternbach, R. A.   *The Psychology of Pain*. Raven Press, New
                    York 1978.
Stubbs, D. A.,   'Back pain research', *Nursing Times* (14 May
    et al.   1981), pp. 857.
Swerdlow, M.   'The value of clinics for the relief of chronic
                    pain', *J. Med. Eth.*, 4 (1978), pp. 117–18.
Twycross, R.   'Principles and practice of the relief of pain
                    in terminal cancer', The Postgraduate
                    Centres, repr. from *Update*, 13 (1972).
                    'Pain and Analgesics', *Current Medical
                    Research and Opinion*, 5:7 (1978),
                    pp. 497–505.
                    'Control of pain', *J. Roy. Coll. Physicians*, 18:1
                    (1984), pp. 32–9.
Waddell, G.   'An approach to backache', *Br. J. Hosp.
                    Med.* (September 1982).
Walker, A. E.   'Somatotopic localization of spinothalamic
                    and secondary trigeminal tract in
                    mesencephalon', *Arch. Neurol. & Psychiatry*,
                    48 (1942), pp. 884–9.
Walsh, T. D., and   'Hospice care: the treatment of pain in
    Saunders, C.   advanced cancer', in *Pain and the Cancer
                    Patient*, ed. M. Zimmerman, P. Drings and
                    G. Wagner, Recent Results in Cancer
                    Research, vol 89. Springer-Verlag, Berlin
                    1984.
Wilson, J. F.   'Behavioral preparation for surgery: benefit
                    or harm?', *J. Behav. Med.*, 4 (1981)
                    pp. 79–100.
Yates, J. W., et al. 'Religion in patients with advanced cancer',
                    Med. & Ped. Oncol., 9 (1981), pp. 121–8.

4

Children and Pain

Instinctive and absolute faith which is strong enough to suppress pain is one of the most beautiful characteristics of children.

Ogilvie and Thomson (1950)

Pain is a fing that hurts.

Sally, aged 9 (1985)

The problem of children's pain is a most complex one, and there appears to be a dearth of systematic research dealing with the subject. There is no firm evidence on which to base the assumption that neonates (newborn) and young children are less sensitive to pain than are adults. In the past it was thought that children could not feel it with the same intensity that adults did, but research has proved this to be a misconception. In his study of children aged between five and eighteen Haslam (1969) observed that the younger the child, the more susceptible he was to pain. Further studies by Beyer et al. (1983), Eland and Anderson (1977) and Mather and Mackie (1983) show that pain in children is undertreated to an even greater extent than pain in adults. At a CIBA Foundation seminar (1985) it was reported with surprise that:

some surgery and certain invasive procedures in neonates are carried out with only minimal anaesthesia and analgesia in some hospitals in Britain, Europe, and America . . . on the assumption that because preterm and even term infants have no memory of pain they are probably not capable of discriminating painful from other stimuli, and because anaesthetic agents may have adverse effects on

71

the cardiovascular and respiratory systems they are best avoided.

The likelihood was expressed that the neonate and possibly the foetus is capable of 'feeling' considerably more than is widely appreciated.

Childhood experiences of pain can prove the most critical determinants of future responses to pain. How young children react to pain will vary considerably, depending upon their age and level of emotional maturity. Birth order can affect a child's response to pain. First-born and only children often appear more anxious than others when anticipating pain as they will have little opportunity of observing pain experiences in brothers and sisters. Such factors, among others, determine the child's physical and psychological response to pain and trauma, as well as the nature of the illness itself. As they move from one stage of development to another children change considerably in the way they interpret suffering and stress.

AGE-DEPENDENT FACTORS

1. *The toddler* up to two years of age is beginning to gain confidence in himself. He is able to recognise his mother as one who cares for him and supplies his needs, and responds to his cry. He already has a limited vocabulary and an equally restricted concept of pain. He normally enjoys activity, doing things, moving his body, pushing and pulling objects around. His enforced passivity when ill restricts movements as well as the enjoyment and control of his body. His early confidence is being undermined. This impairment of normal physical movements can prove one of the most frustrating of experiences for the young child at this early stage. Anna Freud (1952) notes that toddlers, who have only recently learned to walk stand up stubbornly in their beds for the whole course of even a severe illness.

If the toddler has to be removed from his home environment and admitted to hospital his privacy is invaded and he finds himself in strange and unfamiliar surroundings. He may be experiencing pain for the first time in his life, and as his concept of time is as yet undeveloped he will have little idea when the experience is going to end. This makes him more vulnerable to emotional upset than older children, such are his rather limited resources of strength or reasoning powers. Such expressions as 'Mother will only be away for a short time' or 'She'll be back soon' will do very little to reassure an anxious or fretful two-year-old. It is here and now which is all important. The younger the child the greater the degree of anxiety and distress engendered by the unfamiliarity of the clinical environment of a hospital and its uniformed staff.

2. *Pre-school age*. This is probably the most vulnerable stage of all when pain and distress are experienced. Children between the ages of two and five have great sensitivity, and are more aware of the experience of separation than younger infants, and any painful and intrusive procedures are extremely threatening (Bowlby, 1953; Robertson, 1962). They have a very tenuous sense of reality; they live in a world of fantasy, and many of their painful and unpleasant experiences are interpreted as punishment.

The often violent fantasies of the pre-school child can contribute to frightening images of hospitals and surgery and strangers armed with masks, needles and thermometers. Fantasies can be as real, or more real to the young child, as the world of fact around him. He may feel abandoned, unloved and 'let down' and express his pain and displeasure through withdrawal, temper tantrums, and regressed behaviour such as thumbsucking or bedwetting. Separation anxiety is a phenomenon which causes great stress in children under five and the presence of mother is a safeguard against undue anxiety. A pre-school child might be far more stressed about the fear of separation than the painful procedures themselves, for he is often too young to appreciate their implications. According to Piaget (1952) and Werner (1948), in the fundamental domains of space, time, causality and number children adhere to a logic that is qualitatively different from that of adults. Prelogical thinking is typical of children between two and six years of age.

Their behaviour pattern may possibly follow three well-recognised stages. There will be *protest* when the child does not hesitate to make his real feelings known. He becomes anxious, fretful, angry and often uncooperative. This reaction may last from a few hours to several days. A state of *despair* leads to apathy, depression, inability to play, and the child becomes withdrawn and lethargic and in his docility is often mistakenly seen as 'settling in well' and to be 'no trouble'. Yet these can be disturbing signs of anxiety and if not recognised and help given they can lead on to the third stage, of *detachment* or *denial*. His mood seems to cheer up; he responds with smiles and adopts a far more active role. He attaches himself to anyone who is prepared to help but often remains indifferent or hostile to mother. Although appearing happy his mood is often one of resignation rather than contentment.

Where there is a therapeutic milieu and the child is allowed some personal belongings (toys, teddy bear, slippers, favourite blanket), and is able to relate to other toddlers around, much of the trauma of the experience can be mitigated. The presence of mother does much to prevent emotional problems becoming major concerns, and time must be given for both mother and child to adapt to a situation which to them appears alarming and frightening. If procedures are outlined in words he can understand, with truthful explanations, the child's trust is sustained and he is not taken by surprise, shocked or hurt.

3. *School age.* Although the school-age child still has some of the same separation problems and unrealistic fears as younger children they do not become such a hazard. He is able to retain an image of mother in his mind and so does not experience the strong feelings of 'abandonment' during her absence. Social disruption rather than separation from the family becomes the greater problem. Children between four and twelve years of age can communicate verbally and have an adequate concept of pain. They are able to provide information about their pain, and this enables them to handle their feelings and boost their confidence. A study carried out by Eland (1985) with 172 children in hospital, aged between four and ten years, who were asked to place an X on a body outline to show where they had pain, revealed that 168 correctly placed the X and told the researcher why that specific area hurt. A number of studies have shown that children of all ages are able to describe pain as adequately

as adults. The school-age child is able to cope more adequately with his hospitalisation, and his interest and curiosity in what 'goes on' about him helps him to see himself as more of a partner than a victim. At this age physical limitations become extremely irksome and temper tantrums, outbursts, and assaulting behaviour may be an inevitable consequence. His capacity for abstract thinking remains poorly developed and he is liable to misinterpret what is done to him and/or to other children around him (Pinkerton, 1974).

Fears of injections, incisions, and fantasies of mutilation are very vivid at this age because of ill-conceived ideas. The child can often look upon an injection as an attack, a threat to his body integrity, as well as something that hurts. He is normally unable to relate immediate injection pain to future pain relief. The following question was put by Eland (1977) to a group of children in hospital aged between four and ten: 'Of all things that have ever happened to you, what hurt you the worst?' Out of 119 children interviewed 65 replied, 'A needle.' Many young children prefer to put up with the pain than have an analgesic administered by injection. In the mind of the child, admitting he has a pain means he is going to have further pain!

B.D., aged eleven, when asked his thoughts on pain, wrote: 'When I hear somebody say the word "pain" I think of needles. There are other things that hurt but the main one that I think of are needles . . .' Another young child wrote:

> I went into hospital when I was about five, I don't remember every think, but I know I had to have an injection, my mother went out of the room and all the nurses came in I was very frightened. Then they got the injection ready, and when they put it in me I screamed all the way although I didn't feel any pain because I was to busy screaming.

Of all the various experiences undergone during a period in hospital it is significant to note that the only incident remembered was the injection (Jolley, 1985).

For the preservation of his emotional well-being it is imperative for the school-age child to be given an unhurried explanation of all the painful procedures which might be necessary for his treatment. Such reassurance will safeguard his security and prevent the stresses and fears becoming long-lasting and damaging. He may be angry at himself for being ill or in pain and such feelings will often result in destructive, belligerent and hostile behaviour. Honesty and fairness in the provision of information will avoid much misinterpretation and fantasy. One aspect of the perception of pain that the older school-age child (ten to twelve) experiences is that of the fear of death (Schultz, 1971). Such fear probably increases pain, and pain in turn escalates the anxiety.

4. *Adolescence.* The most common fears of older children who are in pain and undergoing surgery revolve around changes in body image, role changes and their sexuality. Often being forced into a dependent-patient role with their natural boister-ousness curtailed, they become moody and volatile. This stage is described by Pinkerton (1974) as notoriously a period of flux, physiologically, emotionally, and in terms of personal values. The adolescent's fear of the loss of control and of identity is very real and disturbing to him. This struggle with his body-image and self-esteem is particularly stressful should he have to undergo surgery.

Many an adolescent feels he should not cry yet does not have the knowledge and experience of an adult to help him cope with his pain. Often the medical team is impressed by the fortitude displayed by teenagers in the face of a painful illness. Like the younger child the adolescent too is 'afraid of life and afraid of death', and all who are caring for him should be sensitive to any expressions of these fears. Korsch (1975) describes adolescence as 'almost as explosive a stage in growth and development as is the pre-school period . . . an apparently minor issue . . . will assume gigantic proportions'. Under stressful situations adolescents are especially fragile, and one of the character trends is that of rebellion and the need to challenge adult authority.

PARENTAL INVOLVEMENT

Studies by Bowlby (1953, 1960, 1961) have shown how mother-deprivation arising from a young child's admission to hospital contributes to much emotional distress. Bowlby emphasises that a young child should always experience a warm, intimate and continuous relationship with his mother or mother-substitute in which both find satisfaction and enjoyment. Children are most sensitive to the atmosphere surrounding them. A mother's kiss or/and affectionate embrace has much healing power, and such utter trust and faith are often strong enough to suppress pain.

The Ministry of Health published a report of its Central Health Services Council in 1959 under the chairmanship of Sir Harry Platt, entitled *The Welfare of Children in Hospital* (commonly called the Platt Report), which stressed the need for sick children to be treated very differently from adult patients. It acknowledged that anxiety for parents and children is reduced by suitable preparation before admission. It recognised that the presence of parents during painful medical procedures, such as drawing blood, aspirating bone marrow, or having a lumbar puncture, provides the child with 'an emotional anchor'. There is a tendency however for some children to exaggerate their pain when a parent is present, and an over-anxious or sensitive mother can communicate her own anxieties and fears to the child. The parents' own experience of pain can influence the attitude of the child, and their own abnormal anxieties increase the child's perception of pain. Parents should never leave a sick child when he is not looking, for this accentuates his feeling of being abandoned. The presence of a calm reassuring parent can prove a safeguard against excessive anxiety and help alleviate the young child's pain. The younger the child the greater the need for such parental support. Winnicott (1958) observed that 'there is no such thing as a baby, only "a mother and infant" ', implying that without its mother no child is able to develop successfully. Until the age of four it is only the actual presence of the mother that can alleviate the young child's anxiety. Where the natural 'bonding' of the mother to her child is disrupted, later disturbances in parent-child relationships may follow.

Parents should always be encouraged to express feelings of concern, their fears and apprehension, for a mother very quickly learns to interpret the behaviour-manifestations of pain in her offspring. Seeing their children in pain and discomfort arouses feelings of guilt and neglect in many parents' minds and they should be shown not to feel responsible for the pain. Anna Freud (1952) has observed how parents undergo a change of attitude when their children are ill, and react quite differently from normal circumstances. They are apt to experience much emotional pain, and although the majority of parents may wish to be with their children it must be acknowledged that not all are capable emotionally of handling and facing up to the situation.

PERSONALITY STRUCTURE

Young children who have been exposed early in life to traumatic experiences prior to hospital admission are inclined to react to pain and discomfort with a greater degree of stress and anxiety. A study carried out by Levy (1960) on the infant's earliest memory of inoculation noted that after the age of six months a young child will recall certain signal qualities of the experience of being inoculated. He will tend to react fearfully to a needle, white coat, restraint, and to subsequent painful situations. Particularly vulnerable are children with poor personality adjustment, the very sensitive and dependent, and those whose relationships with their parents have become disrupted.

The attitudes of parents towards the child's illness or treatment will very largely determine those of the patient himself. Individual children vary considerably: many seem to take things in their stride, while others have excessive fears suggested by crying, over-activity or passive silent co-operation. Jackson (1951) warns about assuming that a calm exterior poise necessarily indicates freedom from anxiety. 'A concrete show of nonchalance may cover a quaking heart.' The more secure the child is emotionally the more able he is to react to the stress of illness and pain. The importance of adverse life circumstances to the hospitalised child cannot be over-emphasised, for events immediately prior to admission, such as the recent arrival of a new baby, the death of a well-loved grandparent, can be very readily misinterpreted by the child. He may see his hospital admission as abandonment by his parents in favour of the new baby. There may be secret fears that he too will 'disappear' as grandma did. On the whole young children are resilient and cope with trauma in ways that often surprise adults, but careful individual assessment of each child is needed because of the tremendous variation in potential reactions.

PREPARATION AND INFORMATION

Much of the fear and anxiety surrounding the child's pain can be reduced by explaining, whenever it is practicable, why the pain is present, how long it is likely to last and what will probably be done to reduce it. This will naturally depend upon how much information he is capable of assimilating, given his age and level of intelligence. When he is oblivious of what is involved he may fantasise and so associate all kinds of fear-inducing experiences with the procedures. If he does not appear to ask for information it should not be assumed that he does not want to know. It may well be that his fear and apprehension inhibits him from asking. By giving the child explanations in advance he is the more able to mobilise his coping skills in preparation.

The Platt Report made a number of important recommendations to promote the welfare of children in hospital and emphasised the necessity of proper preparation to avoid the risk of emotional disturbances and misconceptions. A study carried out by Vaughan (1957) showed how important it is to tell children in hospital as much as they can appreciate about surgical treatment. Children may have quite bizarre and somewhat frightening ideas, and Vaughan shows that what they are told may be much influenced by their parents' own anxiety. Forty children aged four and a half years and over, who had been admitted to hospital for an eye operation, were interviewed and followed up for six months. Many of them had been told nothing, very little, or even direct lies, by their parents. An eight-year-old boy, moved to a more isolated part of the ward because he was vomiting, was given no reason for this and was extremely miserable. He said he had been 'punished' for being naughty and for being a coward during the operation. Asked about his eye surgery, a boy of six said: 'They take it out, turn it round, and cut it, and put it back!' Another child stated: 'I was one of the lucky ones, I got my own eye back!' The study recommends that to be effective the explanation kit should follow an extremely simple course and the child given full opportunity to express his feelings. 'There is a tendency to think of children, and to speak to them, as though they are either miniature adults at one extreme or uncomprehending animals at the other . . . they require accurate explanations – i.e. accurate in that they fit their own concepts – if they are to reassured.'

In discussing how important the timing of preparation is for children undergoing surgery, Korsch (1975) suggests that those under three years of age need preparation hours ahead of time; for those between three and five years preparation should be given days ahead. Older children, dependent on personality, anxiety level and family patterns, may need a few days to a few weeks. The effectiveness of such preparation and information given by supportive parents and sympathetic and understanding staff is well summed up by Potts (1959): 'Children are such amazing creatures. Tell them in simple words . . . why they have to have an operation, and . . . they will co-operate in a fashion that adults might well emulate. Faith and trust are completely unspoilt when children are dealt with honestly. So little effort, so great the reward.'

Children frequently seem to interpret illness and pain as punishment for wrongdoing, and their negative emotional responses are aroused by feelings of rejection and abandonment. Not only do psychological preparation and stress-point supportive care help the children themselves to experience less stress and trauma but also they support and reassure their parents. Wolfer and Visintainer (1975) found that children who are informed, prepared and have factual information about their hospital treatment express less emotional disturbance and more co-operative behaviour. They also seem to experience far fewer post-hospital adjustment problems. The manner of telling is so very important to the child. He needs to be informed by medical or nursing staff 'who are objective but sensitive, involved but stable . . . and in a tone and manner that assure him that medical personnel care about him and are going to help him get well' (Klinzing and Klinzing, 1977).

The uninhibited child who is not too afraid to ask questions about treatment procedures shows fewer episodes of anxiety than another child who hesitates to ask. By asking questions he is the more able to cope. If he is unable to understand what is happening he naturally becomes anxious and stressful. The key factor appears to be that of communication with the provision of truthful information adapted to the child's level of intellectual ability. Such a concept is well outlined by Becker (1972) who states that when a child is admitted to hospital he should not be seen as just the incidental carrier of a disease that is to be cured. He is not measles, rheumatic fever, asthma or sore throat. Rather he is an impressionable human being and a member of a family which is very interested not only in his blood sugar curve or leucocyte count, but, profoundly, in the person that he is.

ASSESSMENT OF PAIN IN CHILDREN

Pain has a subjective quality that eludes precise definition and so cannot easily be assessed. With children the problem becomes more complicated by having to rely in many instances on non-verbal observations. Infants do experience pain regardless of their inability to express their experience verbally, and with increasing age children experience greater pain. Many children seem to conceal their real feelings when suffering pain by becoming taciturn and withdrawn; they hesitate to express their emotions in order to appear 'brave' and 'tough'. Thus they can readily appear to be pain-free when upon questioning by staff or parents they confess to having pain. Mather and Mackie (1983) found that many children will confide in an independent person not apparently associated with hospital life and pain or pain treatment itself. They relate how one young child was observed lying very pale-faced and quietly in bed with his mother close by, only several hours after undergoing orthopaedic surgery. When the nursing staff inquired he denied he had any pain, but questioned by an independent observer dressed in civilian clothes he wept bitterly, and admitted he had severe pain.

The meaning of the word 'pain' is unknown to very young children, and apart from neglecting to complain they may even deny its existence. Some research has shown that children from four to ten years rarely know the meaning of pain as a word before the age of six. To be asked 'Are you in pain?' or 'Where is the pain?' may therefore prove a rather meaningless question. On the other hand it has already been noted (p. 74) that some children are quite articulate in communicating or describing their pain.

The intensity of pain is often indicated by the physical and emotional reactions of the child, and these may serve as useful guidelines in assessing the importance of pain in the young. Signs of irritability may be one reliable indicator of pain. Unfortunately irritable and crying children can sometimes too easily be labelled as 'spoilt'. Often a child will show he is in pain by crying, screaming, or moaning. Crying is an effective form of communication from infant to caregiver. Studies have been made which classify cries according to the type of distress with which they are associated. One such study by Wolff (1969) described three types of infant cries, hunger, anger and pain. The latter is characterised by (a) a sudden onset of loud crying without preliminary moaning, (b) an initial long cry, and (c) an extended period of breath-holding in expiration after a long cry. The most important characteristic to assess pain appears to be the intensity and duration of the crying.

Two recent studies on infant pain have measured various degrees of crying. Two-day-old infants observed by Owens and Todt (1984) cried consistently within three seconds of a heel lance and continued for an average of three minutes. Heart rate also increased and remained elevated for some three and a half minutes. In another clinical study (Williamson and Williamson, 1983) it was found that infants undergoing circumcision also reacted with crying and an increase in heart rate. There are however some children who appear stoical and do not cry at all. Again crying may or may not indicate physical pain. There may also be emotional pain, and crying may be due to sleeping problems, to fear, to absence of mother, or to the presence of overly anxious parents.

Facial expressions may serve as an indication of various internal states. Izard et al. (1980) observed that in the first half-year of life, the pain of physical distress expression that so often follows medical procedures (for example, inoculation) shows 'brows down and together, nasal root broadened and bulged, eyes tightly closed, and the mouth angular and squarish'. In very young infants the difficult discrimination is not between expressions of pain and sadness but between expressions of pain and anger.

Other physical signs of pain include bodily positioning, holding the involved part, and the clenching of fists. A study by Poznanski (1976) revealed that during circumcision babies in the first few days of life will commonly react with a total body movement. The cries associated with the procedure are usually brief and cease on distraction. Earlier research by McGraw (1945), which investigated the reaction to pin-prick in infants from birth to four years, found that until they were ten days old some infants made no motor response to pin-prick: if however the neonate did react the characteristic response was 'diffuse body movement'. Infants between six months and a year old exhibited 'purposeful withdrawal' of the stimulated limb. By the age of one year infants touched the area of stimulation after the stimulus was withdrawn. In older children fear, frustration, anxiety, loneliness, anger, may be signs of emotional pain expressed in the postoperative stage. It is extremely difficult to differentiate physical pain from various negative experiences after surgical procedures, and not until the child is conscious and the effects of anaesthesia have worn off can physical signs be used to assess and identify pain accurately. If he can be encouraged to help in some of the nursing procedures such as changing dressings it may well cause a less negative affect to be attached to his assessment of proceedings.

As pain is essentially a private experience the problem of interpreting the significance of such reactions is indeed most formidable. Even at a very early stage there are substantial individual differences in how infants react. An additional complication is that anxiety and various emotional factors may augment or distort the child's response to pain. Again a number of young children tend to react to pain in a manner characteristic of their family background. The age of the child, his developmental level, prior experience of pain, advance preparation and information about pain treatments, his birth order and sex, are all contributory factors in determining how he will respond to the experience of pain. If the child says he is in pain he must be taken at his word and his pain acknowledged by medical and nursing staff. He should always be given permission to feel pain. An important aspect of future research regarding pain in infants is the study of the recovery and reorganisation of behaviour after painful procedures.

PSYCHOLOGICAL FACTORS

Psychological factors play a part as a pre-existing cause in the experience of pain in children. Often each child will react in a personal manner depending upon age and family. It is in the parental environment of the family that the child develops his model of interaction and in which he experiments with his knowledge. This is particularly relevant for the preschool child for his whole world revolves around the parental figures. Pain may serve as an ego defence, a symbolic substitute absorbing the attention of the subject and allowing him to protect himself against difficulties and anxieties which probably cause more suffering than the actual pain. From the psychological viewpoint pain can be considered as one of many different ways of reacting to stress and anxiety. Older children often complain of periods of pain for which no evident organic cause can be found. Various studies reveal that these children normally range in age from five to sixteen, and tend to come from families in which the parents are prone to pain. Children can be great 'imitators', and are often able to develop some of the symptoms of painful experiences of their parents.

One of the most common pain complaints in young children is recurrent abdominal and chest pain yet most of these pains do not seem to have an organic basis. Anxiety and other emotional factors play a very important part in causing this sort of pain, and often children with family and/or school problems are affected. Also present are secondary gains in the form of an opportunity to withdraw from difficult and threatening situations. Domestic difficulties can arise from parental quarrels, a father who has over-ambitious expectations of a child, or difficulties at school. The onset of the symptom may also coincide with a particular event or difficult period in the life of the child such as marital, financial or

84

housing problems of the parents. Painful syndromes are familial. Apley (1967, 1971) found that recurrent abdominal pain was observed in one out of nine school children, and only about 5 per cent of children were brought into paediatric clinics for abdominal pain with an organic origin. Such children had a wide variety of emotional problems.

Another common cause of absence from school in older children is a headache. Studies suggest that headaches tend to occur three years later than stomach pains and reach a maximum occurrence at twelve years of age. In a number of subjects it has been found that as well as family and school difficulties they also have a parent or a relative affected by headaches, and are usually children over-protected by their parents.

It is to be noted that in the majority of instances a psychological cause does not signify that the child is feigning his pain and discomfort; he is really suffering and if parents and physician do not profer adequate care and attention disorders of emotional origin can develop into organic diseases. Although entirely of psychological origin the pain is real to the child concerned.

The child's experiences with pain and his reactions to it will serve to influence the individual's response to pain in later life. Familial and individual attitudes will colour his concepts about pain and affect all his thoughts about suffering.

Apley, J.	'The child with recurrent abdominal pain', *Ped. Clin. North Am.*, 14:1 (1967).
Apley, J., et al.	'Pupillary reaction in children with recurrent abdominal pain', *Arch. Dis. Child.*, 46 (1971) p. 337.
Becker, R. D.	'Therapeutic approaches to psychopathological reactions to hospitalization', *Inter. J. Child Psychotherapy*, 1 (1972), pp. 65–97.
Beyer, J. E., et al.	'Patterns of postoperative analgesic use with adults and children following cardiac surgery', *Pain*, 17 (1983), pp. 71–81.

Bowlby, J.   'Some pathological processes set in train by early mother-child separation', *J. Ment. Science*, 99 (1953), pp. 265–72.
Child Care and the Growth of Love. Penguin, London 1953.
'Separation anxiety', *Inter. J. Psychoanal.*, 41 (1960), pp. 89–113.
'Childhood mourning and its implications for psychiatry', *Amer. J. Psychiatry*, 118 (1961), pp. 481–98.

CIBA Foundation   'Can a fetus feel pain?', *Brit. Med. J.*, 291 (2 November 1985), pp. 1220–1.

Cromwell, F. S.   (ed.) *Occupational Therapy and the Patient with Pain*. Haworth, New York 1984.

Eland, J. M.   'The child who is hurting', *Seminars in Oncology Nursing*, 1:2 (1985), pp. 116–22.

Eland, J. M., and   'The Experience of pain in children', in A.
Anderson, J. E.   Jacox (ed.), *Pain: a source book for nurses and other health professionals*. Little, Brown, Boston 1977.

Freud, A.   'The role of bodily illness in the mental life of children', in *The Psychoanalytical Study of the Child*, VII (1952), pp. 69–82.

Haslam, D. R.   'Age and the perception of pain', *Psychonomic Sci.*, 15 (1969), pp. 86–7.

Izard, C. E., et al.   'The young infant's ability to produce discrete emotion expressions', *Develop. Psychol.*, 16 (1980), pp. 132–40.

Jackson, K.   'Psychological preparation as a method of reducing the emotional trauma of anesthesia in children', *Anesthesiology*, 12 (1951), p. 293.

Jolley, J.   'Timmy goes to hospital', *Nursing Times* (27 March 1985).

Klinzing, D. R.,   *The Hospitalized Child*. Prentice-Hall, New
and D. G.   Jersey 1977.

Korsch, B. M.   'The child and the operating room', *Anesthesiology*, 43 (2) (1975), p. 251.

Levy, D. M.   'The infant's earliest memory of inoculation: a contribution to public health procedures', *J. Genet. Psychol.*, 96:3 (1960).

McGraw, M. B.	*The Neuromuscular Maturation of the Human Infant*. Hafner, New York 1945.
Mather, L., and Mackie, J.	'The incidence of postoperative pain in children', *Pain*, 15 (1983), pp. 271–82.
Michel, T. H.	(ed.) *Pain: international perspectives in physical therapy*. Churchill Livingstone, Edinburgh 1985.
Owens, M. E., and Todt, E. H.	'Pain in infancy: neonatal reaction to a heel lance', *Pain*, 20 (September 1984), pp. 76–86.
Piaget, J.	*The Child's Conception of Physical Causality*. Kegan Paul, London 1952.
Pinkerton, P.	'Preventing psycho trauma in childhood', in *Modern Trends in Anaesthesia*, ed. J. Rees and C. T. Gray. Churchill Livingstone, Edinburgh (1981), pp. 1–18. *Childhood Disorder: a psychosomatic approach*. Crosby Lockwood Staples, London 1974.
Platt, H.	*The Welfare of Children in Hospital*, Platt Report, Min. Health. HMSO, London 1959.
Potts, W. J.	*The Surgeon and the Child*. Saunders, Philadelphia 1959.
Poznanski, E. O.	'Chidren's reactions to pain: a psychiatrist's perspective', *Clinical Pediatrics*, 15:12 (1976), pp. 114–19.
Robertson, J.	*Young Children in Hospitals*. Basic Books, New York 1958. (ed.) *Hospitals and Children*. Gollancz, London 1962.
Schultz, N.	'How children perceive pain', *Nursing Outlook*, 19 (1971), p. 670.
Vaughan, G. F.	'Children in Hospital', *Lancet*, 1 (1957), p. 1117.
Visintainer, M. A., and Wolfer, J. A.	'Psychological preparation for surgical pediatric patients: the effect on children's and parents' stress responses and adjustments', *Pediatrics*, 56 (2) (1975), p. 187.
Werner, H.	*Comparative Psychology of Mental Development*. Science Editions, New York 1948.

Williamson, P. S., and M. L. — 'Physiologic stress reduction by a local anesthetic during newborn circumcision', *Pediatrics*, 71 (January 1983), pp. 36–40.

Winnicott, D. W. — *Through Paediatrics to Psychoanalysis.* Tavistock, London 1958.

Wolff, P. H. — 'The natural history of crying and other vocalizations in early infancy', in B. Foss (ed.), *Determinants of Infant Behavior*, vol IV (Methuen, London 1969), pp. 81–115.

5

Attitudes to Pain

Pain makes man think.

      John Patrick, *The Teahouse of the August Moon* (1953)

He must be wicked to deserve such pain.

Robert Browning, *Childe Roland to the Dark Tower Came* (1855)

Attitudes to pain will vary according to social and cultural backgrounds, the classification of the disease which causes the pain, as well as the personality characteristics of the patient. For many patients their pain is a private experience and there is a reluctance to express personal feelings. There are those who are more expressive of their pain in the presence of a doctor or nurse, while others feel more free to 'let go' with family or friends. Different personalities naturally react in various ways.

ATTITUDE OF THE CARER

Professional carers are trained to respond objectively to sickness and the pain and discomfort that often accompany it. However it must be borne in mind that the carers are first of all human beings, and subject to the same pressures of guilt and inadequacy as other people. The following comments taken from a survey (1985) conducted by the author are self evident:

The doctor does not – regrettably perhaps – have the intimate contact with the patient in pain that the nurse has, nor does he usually have the time or opportunity to supervise, minute by minute, hour by hour, the relief of the pain. (Senior Registrar)

The doctor subscribes appropriate regimens for the pain whose cause, nature and severity he thinks he understands and trusts that this is implemented by members of the nursing staff. (Senior House Officer)

If I am very truthful with myself, I find it difficult to nurse people who are in great pain (physical or emotional). Pain causes people to become irritable, edgy, restless, short-tempered, and more difficult to communicate with. Thus to nurse someone in pain requires greater patience and understanding, and even insight into the root of the pain and how best it can be alleviated. (2nd year nursing student)

Nursing a patient with severe pain is not an easy task for me, especially if the pain is prolonged. I must keep the patient's welfare in mind and try and make the patient feel comfortable as far as possible, and try and relieve anxiety and pain by the nursing procedures and especially by the way I present myself to the patient. (1st year nursing student)

It is a challenge to me, although it taxes me emotionally. (1st year nursing student)

Both medical and nurse training have concentrated to a large extent on the *cure* of disease which 'has in general diverted attention, thought, research and training away from the problems, such as severe pain or nausea, of those patients with diseases which have yet to be curable' (Melzack and Wall, 1982).

The carers' own attitudes to pain and suffering are important factors. Their inability to 'cure' may lead to a sense of failure, and a consequent loss of interest in the patient. There may also be a tendency to infer less pain than a patient actually experiences. Those who are customarily involved with patients in pain may feel so overwhelmed that there may be a tendency to protect themselves by denying it, or by becoming so familiar with it that they 'turn it off':

It is essential I feel that each patient is nursed individually so that we don't become blasé about it – which is difficult, especially on a surgical ward, where you've seen patients in pain then later recovered: it's then all too easy to just tell the patient that the pain is to be expected, and will eventually go. (3rd year nursing student)

It is a matter of inadequacy of time and facilities rather than inadequacy of knowledge and drugs. The treatment of one person with persistent pain is almost a full-time job – at least until a satisfactory treatment regimen has been established. This is where the hospice movement comes right into its own. (Consultant Anaesthetist)

In some ways one would regard persistent pain as failure. What am I going to do about it? If my simple drug regimens have failed then I would consult with those who are more experienced in this particular field. (Registrar)

There may be a tendency for staff to value stoicism and admire patients with strong will-power and those who have the ability to 'put up with things', Nurses have a direct and prolonged contact with those who suffer, and are associated with the intimate details of physical pain and various distressing psychological attributes of illness. In their daily work both physician and nurse repeatedly encounter suffering and distress, both physical and psychological, and are called to apply their skill in attempting to alleviate it.

Those who have never experienced severe pain themselves often find it difficult to empathise with someone else's pain. On the other hand, a nurse or young doctor who has been through a painful experience may be especially sensitive to the suffering of another. Such identification can make a significant difference to the response, as illustrated by the following:

Since undergoing minor surgery and fracturing my radius last year, surgical and orthopaedic patients will be looked upon in a new light . . . There is nothing more annoying than being told that, 'It shouldn't hurt now, come on, you've only had a – . (1st year nursing student)

Having experienced hospital from the patient's side several times, I feel I have a better idea of the importance of occupation, friends, company and general antidotes to lone-liness and depression! (1st year nursing student)

I underwent rather painful surgery to have my gall-bladder out last year and I feel I can now experience other people's pain far more sympathetically. I doubt whether I would have the same kind of fellow-feeling and understanding if I hadn't recently experienced such pain and discomfort myself. (Senior House Officer)

I think if you can recall any pain you have suffered that it helps towards putting yourself in the patient's position . . . (2nd year student nurse)

Feelings of sympathy often lead to increased contact with the patient:

Something happens to you when you're with patients you feel a lot for. I think it's like a wave of gentleness or tenderness. It sweeps over you when you care. I suppose I show it in my voice and hands. I know that inside I feel warm and soft, I'm sure I do something to express that feeling. (Davitz and Davitz, 1975)

There are many patients who don't realise how demoral-ising chronic pain is. They can become very ill through pain itself. In some instances they become so used to it that they don't realise how much pain they are in. This makes assessment extremely difficult. They forget what normal life is like. (Professor of Surgery)

This is borne out by one patient who remarked, 'Throughout the eighteen years I suffered with pain I got so used to pain that it was hard to believe when there were odd days when I suffered no pain at all. Sometimes I thought I imagined until I had a painless day.'

The stress of being rather overwhelmed on occasions by the suffering of patients can influence attitudes and affect relationships:

I am often aware that prolonged and repeated exposure to patients who are in pain reduces my sensitivity and makes me rather cold and detached. I feel guilty afterwards if I have been terse and kept conversation to a minimum, and try and make up for my negative feelings. (Surgical Registrar)

I pride myself that I can cope with most of the conditions on the Ward, but when I see some of the patients in acute pain I realise that with all my nursing experience, underneath I'm just a rather soft emotional person – with all that that entails. I want to be with them – yet if I'm honest I don't want to be with them! (Staff Nurse)

Medication can be given to relieve the physical pain of a patient but many a carer feels rather inadequate when having to deal with mental or emotional distress. The following responses demonstrate some of the difficulties involved and how best they can be resolved:

In the past nurses, if seen to be spending time talking to their patients, were told to get on with their work – fortunately we now have far more enlightened views and realise that talking to patients – helping them to talk to us – *is* work, and often hard work at that! It is extremely satisfying and rewarding but in some instances it can be very emotionally draining. (Nursing Officer)

It can be very tiring, and extreme patience must be exercised and time taken to talk to a patient who is mentally disturbed, and I find this very difficult to deal with. I am much happier and feel more secure when I can do things to and for a patient. You see some results of your nursing then, but with psychological pain, what do you say? What do you do? (2nd year nursing student)

I can cope with seeing people in physical pain fairly well. However, I find it quite difficult to relieve a patient's emotional pain . . . I find the best thing to do when faced with a person in emotional or mental pain is to simply listen to them. It usually makes them feel better and more relaxed, despite my feeling I have done nothing to help them. (1st year nursing student)

I find this among my most difficult tasks – to try and spend time – when time is so precious – unravelling some of their problems, putting them straight on some strange and bizarre ideas they've probably picked up from other people

– often from other patients who have described their treatments and operations and the after-effects! So many want a listening ear and reassurance. If I've been able to gain their confidence I normally get somewhere in the end – at least I hope I do! (Ward Sister)

Unfortunately there doesn't seem to be lot of time to sort out what is really causing the patient to feel depressed or emotionally upset. You can't deal with the problem in a matter of minutes. It may be necessary to call in one of the other disciplines, such as the chaplain or social worker. It is very difficult not to let your emotions make you less professional. (2nd year nursing student)

Such emotional pain can be very frustrating for any nurse, no matter how experienced, when she senses her helplessness in attempting to support and comfort the patient. It can be equally draining if not more than seeing a patient in physical pain. (3rd year nursing student)

If I can keep myself from avoiding it, ideally, I like to get them to talk with me, tell me how the pain feels and where, then perhaps *together* we can choose the best course of action to alleviate it. (2nd year nursing student)

The preference of staff for dealing with physical problems often inhibits those in pain from mentioning their psychological and emotional problems. Maguire (1984) established that the knowledge of the social and psychological problems of patients is seriously deficient, and is unrecognised in up to 50 per cent of physically ill patients. Nurses generally find it easier to concentrate on physical care and physical tasks. Difficult questions asked by patients can be threatening: 'Is it cancer?', 'Why me?', 'How long have I got?' If such emotive questions are avoided serious consequences can follow, because it means the patient's care plan will be based on inadequate data. The ability to sympathise and understand a patient's psychological problems, and so help to allay anxiety and fear, is just as important as actual treatment for the relief of pain. Diers et al. (1972) conclude that the nursing approach which takes into account the 'whole patient' is more likely to produce pain relief and the effect of nursing is greater than the effect of medication alone in providing pain relief.

It is just here that the art as well as the science of both medicine and nursing can be demonstrated.

The *age* of the patient appears to have little bearing on nurses' inferences of physical pain although for some it does seem to be a crucial factor in determining their attitude. In the survey (1985) undertaken by the author it was found that nurses consistently seem to infer greater suffering in very young patients, in those of their own age, and in the very old:

> Perhaps my sympathies are more aroused by a very young child in pain, because of the fear that often accompanies it – not knowing or fully understanding why they are in pain. (2nd year nursing student)

> I feel more sympathetic towards children as they do not understand pain whereas adults are 'used' to the feeling and can somewhat accept it. (1st year nursing student)

> I possibly feel more sympathetic towards a younger person because I tend to compare myself more with them. Easier to understand what the patient is going through if they are approximately the same age as yourself. However the same may be true of someone my parent's age, for example. (3rd year nursing student)

> Often, if the patient is of a similar age or younger the pain is 'seen' more, or perhaps experienced more. Also at the other end of the scale, the old people. (3rd year nursing student)

> Elderly patients are far more tolerant towards their pain. Indeed many almost feel that they should have pain! It's part and parcel of old age! (Ward Sister)

> We tend to be more sympathetic and alert to the pains of the very young and the very old patients than with those in middle-age. We expect them to cope better. (1st year student nurse)

Although the *sex* of the patient does not generally seem to influence the attitude of the carers, there appears to be more awareness of the 'tough image' of the male:

> As a society we probably place pressure on men to 'prove themselves' as strong and self-willed when in pain but I

feel for them as much as I do for any woman. (4th year nursing student)

I find that women express their pain more openly and thus it is essential to listen to male patients carefully and ask them about their pain. There is a tendency to regard it as more 'socially acceptable' for women to complain more of pain than men. (2nd year nursing student)

I feel men often behave too stoically. (1st year nursing student)

Men do tend to try and keep a 'stiff-upper-lip'. I find it quite distressing when men cry. (1st year nursing student)

Attitudes can be influenced by the *specific illness* of the patient. Patients suffering from a painful condition, cancer, or a terminal illness arouse much concern:

If the patient is dying or seriously ill, my sympathies are more aroused than if the patient has just undergone a 'routine' operation, though clearly the pain to each patient is equally real. (2nd year nursing student)

If it is an illness that I know is associated with a great deal of pain, then perhaps I can empathise more with that patient. However I take all complaints of pain as being genuine. (2nd year nursing student)

I suppose as nurses we can use the argument that the patient's illness is to be expected to produce pain as a way of coping. For instance, we might expect someone with arthritis to be in constant pain, and so we feel that the patient should also expect to be in pain and should therefore be better able to 'grin and bear it'. I try not to become hardened to these people's experiences however little emphasis we place on the importance of their pain as a profession. (4th year nursing student)

There are very naturally feelings of helplessness, failure, anger, distress and frustration when the professional carer is unable to relieve pain:

Frustrated, very frustrated. Incompetent – I feel as if I *should* be able to help this person. (1st year student nurse)

I feel guilty, angry, inadequate, and occasionally, when exasperated, indifferent. (1st year nursing student)

What many people do not realise is that it is painful *for us* to see a patient suffer and be unable to offer relief. (Staff Nurse)

I question why the pain has not been relieved – is there something else I or others can do? What is wrong with my care because I have failed to relieve the patient's pain problem? (1st year nursing student)

There is an awful feeling of 'helplessness' when a patient still is in pain. Depending on the reasons I may feel angry – perhaps if other health-care team members have neglected the patient's needs. And there is a feeling of guilt – often when the patient asks for more relief and has to wait until the next dose can be given. (3rd year nursing student)

Being so frustrated at my own impotence to alleviate the pain I often find I am denying it and inwardly blaming the patient for 'putting it on'. (Senior Registrar)

Similar emotions are also aroused when a nurse has to carry out procedures which she knows will cause the patient further pain, although such negative feelings are somewhat modified by the assurance that the nursing duties are being performed for the eventual benefit of the patient – for example, the prevention of pressure-sores:

I think my attitude varies – if the outcome of the procedures can be seen to be essential for the well-being of the patient, it makes it easier, and if I am able to tell the patient this – and he/she understands (without making false promises). But there are often patients who for some reason or another may not be able to understand or communicate adequately (babies, very young children). Whenever possible I try to explain fully to the patient what I'm going to do. (3rd year nursing student)

If one can understand the rationale behind it then one feels justified and takes precautions to keep pain to a minimum. (1st year nursing student)

I try my best to be honest about what I am doing to do, how long I think it will take, etc. I try to encourage them to see a good outcome at the end of the procedure. (1st year nursing student)

Information and explanation are seen as very necessary requisites:

Full explanations of the process I feel are essential, and the nurse must listen to the patients' feelings and fears. (2nd year nursing student)

If possible I ensure that the procedure is carried out soon after the latest dose of pain-killers. I think one has to explain that the procedure will hurt, and be as gentle and careful as possible, stopping when the patient shows signs of pain. (3rd year nursing student)

Both doctors and nurses often have personal biases and preconceived ideas about how much pain a patient should be experiencing with each disease entity. In these circumstances the patient may feel that his statement of pain is not being accepted or appreciated by the medical and nursing staff, and/or that he is being 'diagnosed' a malingerer eager to gain attention, or someone who is 'always complaining':

So readily can we brand those who are in constant pain 'neurotic'. Breast pain (mastalgia) might be a typical example. It can be perceived from a traditional surgical view that pain in the breast is largely an expression of psychoneurosis, but most patients have a physiological or pathological basis for their breast pain, and differ greatly from those with recognised psychoneurosis. They deserve an appropriate diagnostic and therapeutic approach. (Lecturer in Surgery)

Nurses have certain expectations regarding patients who have every reason to complain of their pain and those whom they consider to be over-acting. So easily can it be thought or expressed, 'You can't possibly be in pain – you've already had your pain-killers!' If complaints are unwarranted the nurse naturally becomes irritated and annoyed, and there is a tendency to avoid the patient. 'I feel I know who is sick and who is making a noise. Then I realise I treat people who

I feel are really sick differently from the way I do people who are just making a noise.' 'When I don't feel a patient is really in pain . . . and he keeps calling for a nurse, I get annoyed. I mean, there are patients who really need me.' On reflection many a nurse reports a sense of guilt and is eager to 'make up' for any seeming neglect: 'I feel guilty because I know the patient is sick and maybe not responsible for his actions. I can't help not liking the patient but I also feel guilty. Then I go to the patient's room and try to make it up to him' (Davitz and Davitz, 1975).

Such attitudes bear out the earlier statement that members of the caring professions who tend those in pain are but people and therefore prone to the same emotional feelings and pressures as others. In general both physicians' and nurses' attitudes are directly or indirectly influenced by their own psychological 'make-up', as well as their acquired beliefs about pain and suffering. The carer's own values should not be imposed upon the patient, for then there will always be the tendency to be judgmental.

ATTITUDE OF THE FAMILY

Those who have to watch loved ones suffer and be alongside them during periods of pain are often immediately overcome with feelings of impotence and helplessness. The indignities of pain and suffering cause much mental and emotional distress to those who watch and wait:

> Pain that is uncontrolled leads to a death without grace and dignity. It destroys the person who suffers it, breaks the family who witness it and brands the staff who pass by on the other side. (Mother of a patient with cancer [Raiman, 1986])

'If only we could do something' is a common cry:

> We feel so helpless. Nothing we seem to do appears to help. It's cruel having to sit here hour after hour and see A. suffering like this. Sometimes I wish he would just go – he'd be at peace then and out of his pain. (Son of elderly patient who had a large tumour removed from rear of left eye).

99

It's the utter helplessness that gets you! What can you do? What can you say? You can only sit and think and cry. Your hands are tied – everything seems tied. (Wife of patient with gangrene of left foot)

This natural desire is undermined with feelings of guilt. The family may reflect with regret on events which might have happened in the past, and look back to any unhappy inter-personal relationships within the family circle:

As I sit here by the beside I think – think too much probably. I go back over our lives together. We've had a happy time – it's not always been a rosy picture and I wish I had done more. He hasn't been well over the past five/six years yet we've struggled on and sort of pretended all was well. It's been a dreadful strain and I feel drained. I should have *made him* go to the doctor's months ago but kept on putting it off. I shall always blame myself for that. (Wife of elderly patient who underwent abdomino-perineal excision of rectum)

We've never been a united family – always seem to be squabbling. J. was out of work and the boys don't get on with their step-father. We never bothered with my brothers – no one's perfect, I know, but I feel if only we'd been happier together. It's all too late now! – and I shall live to regret it. (Wife of patient with carcinoma of stomach)

Guilt sometimes becomes readily projected on to members of the caring team who are criticised for not doing all that they might to help in the situation:

You'd think in a new hospital like this they wouldn't let people suffer. The doctors don't seem to be able to do much about L.'s case and the nurses seem far too young and inexperienced to understand. Let's have back the old days, I say – at least you knew who was who then. They don't seem to have any time for patients these days, only get them out of hospital as soon as possible – off their hands! There doesn't seem the caring about there used to be. I wish L. was still in St B's hospital – he got on well there. (Sister of patient with renal colic)

Denial and withdrawal are common symptoms developed in

order to counteract feelings of guilt and inadequacy. There is an inner and conflicting tension to approach the bedside and to withdraw from the scene. Sometimes the family may feel too constrained by the very hospital atmosphere or environment to offer the patient support and comfort:

> Sometimes I can't seem to get near enough to him. He doesn't seem to be mine any longer – I feel he's become hospital property, and I'm just a stranger appearing on the scene from time to time. There seems a barrier – an invisible barrier – which comes between us. I'm his wife and yet I get this awful feeling of being just a shadow, someone on the side-lines, who has to ask permission to see him. I'd love to cuddle him and get close but somehow I feel I mustn't, so I just sit and hold his hand. I'm not always sure he even knows I'm here. (Wife of patient with trigeminal neuralgia)

There will often be anger which is a response to a threatening situation and based on anxiety. Open and free expressions of it by members of the family can do much to relieve their tenseness and help restore a sense of self-control. Such anger is not a single response but a series of reactions comprising frustration and unfulfilled expectations; it is an assertive protection against feelings of helplessness, and is often related to guilt. Anger can be projected against both things and persons, for example, the hospital ward is too noisy, the bed too hard, the staff not caring enough, and God himself has deserted them.

There may be confusion in the minds of the family if they do not understand why certain procedures are or are not being carried out to alleviate their relative's pain and discomfort:

> I can't understand it! Why don't they give him something to get rid of his pain. You'd think he could have an injection or something. They're supposed to be so clever these days but I'm beginning to have my doubts. I wish they'd spend more money on cancer research than on all those nuclear weapons. Why don't they give him some pain-killers? I've had a word with Sister but she's always busy, and I haven't seen a doctor round for days! (Close friend of patient with carcinoma of bronchus)

101

Naturally there is much worry and concern. Will the outcome be fatal? Are they telling me everything?

> I remember when D. was very ill, we had to pretend she didn't have cancer. I'm worried stiff J. has got it now. I thought he was getting better, and they said he'd probably be home in four/five days – he's been here two weeks already. It's the doctors who recommended he had this operation – I wasn't too keen – I knew what happened to D. I honestly don't know where to turn. If he goes and leaves me what am I going to do? Who'll look after Gran? I want to have a word with the surgeon but to be truthful I'm afraid it will only be bad news. (Wife of patient who underwent surgery for removal of gastric ulcer)

There are occasions when such adverse circumstances seem to bind families together. In periods of acute stress and concern inhibitions seem to dissolve and a degree of openness and bonding emerge:

> I must be honest and say that over these past few weeks N. and I have been closer than for many a long day. It's been a rather wonderful experience and a real eye-opener for me. N. was never a one to share his feelings – rather cold emotionally but I understood him and loved him. He was always rather shy and reserved even with me. Our friends used to tease me about him. But since his illness and my being here with him, often alone and in the quiet, things seem to have changed – we are far more open with each other these days and we've had long intimate chats we would never think of having before. Yes, I can honestly say we've grown closer together since N.'s been like this. (Wife of patient suffering from carcinoma of prostate gland)

Family members, estranged in the past, are now ready to 'rally round' and lend support, putting 'old scores' behind them:

> My sisters have been wonderful. We never had much to do with one another. We went our separate ways and brought up our families independent of each other. We've never been really close – I don't think my friends knew I had four sisters. But since B.'s illness they've 'turned up

trumps'. They've stayed with me here in hospital and this meant all the world to me. B.'s been in a lot of pain but I'm sure it's done her the world of good seeing us all one big happy family again. They've been wonderful and I shan't forget them! (Husband of patient with herpes zoster shingles over right eye)

Should the patient be at home and in pain there may arise resentment between siblings or other family members on account of the sick person 'getting all the attention' and sympathy. Such negative feelings are frequently sensed by the patient himself and liable to cause him greater discomfort both physically and emotionally.

Where there is no family support or the husband/wife is alone in hospital, to watch and attempt to comfort, the experience can be very emotionally traumatic and draining:

We seem to be in two separate, water-tight worlds P. and I. I can't talk to him and there's no one around to talk to either. They're all so busy and I feel really frightened here all on my own. I know the nurses would come if I asked them but they're all so busy and they've got their work to do, and I know they're very short-staffed on this ward. There were only two nurses on all last night. It's being so much on my own that frightens me – I keep the door open so I can see people passing. (Wife of terminally ill patient)

Often there can be a sense of guilt, 'survival guilt', at being the healthy one, while another member of the family is suffering and in pain. Such feelings are coupled with the desire to take the place of the patient:

Why should B. have to have all the pain and here am I getting off so lightly. I've been one of those fortunate ones – never had a day's illness in my life while B. has had years of suffering. He doesn't deserve it – I often feel I'm the one to deserve it. I haven't been all I might have been to him. Often I just want to put myself in B.'s place and suffer instead of him – take some of his pain away. I'd willingly bear anything for him. (Wife of patient after myocardial infarction)

The great courage shown and the sincere gratitude expressed

by many a family affords much encouragement to members of the hospital staff who are ministering to the patient, and provides them with an added zest to their vocation as carers:

> I can't speak too highly of the staff here. They're real angels, those nurses. I shall never be able to repay them. Every time I come to visit M. tells me how good they are to him. They always seem to have time for a chat and that means a lot, I can tell you. I shall never forget Mr B. for his kindness too – he's the one who did the operation. He's seen M. every day and also sees that he gets constant relief from his pain – he's assured me that they're doing their best to make him symptom-free. (Sister-in-law of patient after cholecystectomy, removal of gall-bladder)

The assurance that the patient is being remembered by the local community or is on the prayer-list of his church gives many a family additional support and stimulus. They are not alone in the situation but are being strengthened by those around them, and being made conscious of belonging to a caring fellowship or congregation.

If the family are able to remain calm and confident, assured that all that can be done is being done to control the pain, their very presence will have a reassuring effect upon their loved one and help much to allay the pain experience. 'What is good in any painful experience', wrote C. S. Lewis (1940), 'is for the sufferer, his submission to the will of God, and for the spectators, the compassion aroused and the acts of mercy to which it leads.'

ATTITUDE OF THE PATIENT

There will be as many attitudes to pain as there are patients, for each sufferer is a unique individual. A hospital ward of twenty patients may be labelled 'medical' or 'surgical', yet there will be twenty different sets of emotions and attitudes, ranging from feelings of dejection, abandonment, punishment, submission to God's will, 'the devil at work', defiance, to challenge and courage. Copp (1974) interviewed some 148 patients in five hospitals and in all stages of pain experience to learn what pain meant to them and how they coped.

Some sixteen patients (11 per cent) thought of their pain and suffering as a challenge and assumed there would be 'emotional and spiritual' effects on their future-life. Thirty-three patients (22 per cent) described struggling and overcoming their suffering, but fifteen (10 per cent) were quick to blame themselves and perceived their pain as weakness on their own part. It is interesting to note that nineteen of the patients (13 per cent) conceived of their pain as punishment. Almost a third of those interviewed, thirty-nine patients (26 per cent), reported value in their experience of pain. Naturally they would have preferred to have avoided their suffering, yet they saw value in it as an opportunity for creative expression, self-searching, and self-testing, encouraging appreciation of what patients less fortunate than themselves had gone through, and permitting identification with others who had suffered. For the majority pain and suffering had strong religious connotations.

The typically British attitude to pain is to adopt the 'stiff-upper-lip' approach, 'It's just one of those things!' Strong values are placed on bravery, endurance and the ability to bear pain with silent fortitude. Many patients are encountered who feel it is 'right and proper' to bear as much pain as they can before they ask for an analgesic. Attempts are made to ignore or conceal their pain from others. Not only do they believe they are betraying their Christian faith or beliefs by 'complaining', but also they do not want to create any impression of letting their family or friends down by giving any intimation of being in pain, or of being a nuisance to nursing staff. 'I feared disappointing my friends and relations as well as being labelled a "difficult patient" by the nursing staff,' remarked one patient after recovering from rather painful surgery.

Patients often feel guilty or ashamed of attitudes such as these, so much so that their personal evaluation of their behavioural reactions may create more anxiety than the actual pain itself. They feel they are failing to live up to other people's and indeed their own personal expectations. A high pain threshold is associated in the patient's mind with courage, and moral judgments can unconsciously be made by the carers. The brave uncomplaining patient is often complimented and offered sympathy, while those who appear

105

intolerant of seemingly minor discomfort or pain are branded as 'a nuisance' or the 'always complaining' type.

It is apparent that social stigma can become attached to complaints about pain (Jacox and Stewart, 1973). Such an attitude is borne out by such expressions as: 'I rarely discuss it unless someone asks me, I'm not one of those hypochondriac types' or 'No one likes a complainer.'

On occasions there will be conditional replies: 'It all depends on who is asking me about it.' Jacox found that two-thirds of the patients she asked about their pain were eager not to show when they experienced it. They made comments such as: 'I know that it's not going to last for ever, and that it will pass' or 'I ignore it as much as I can.'

Some patients remark that although their pain does distress them they try not to make it obvious and keep it to themselves: 'All you can do is just lie there and stick it out. There's not much point in putting on a big show.' 'I'm just as tough as the rest of them!'

Often people in pain do not seem to have the ability to think beyond their pain. A number of patients are not prepared to mention it until it is severe, and some may not say anything at all. There is also much prejudice among some patients about the use of pain-relieving drugs, and pain is seen as a weakness on their part. Hayward (1980) in his study found that there were many patients who considered that such drugs were much better done without, and that there was a general preference to 'stick it out', rather than give in to what was regarded as weakness and ask for relief of their pain. There is a common tendency to see pain as a sort of trial – 'These things are sent to test us' – and by such stoicism triumphing over it unaided is therefore to become a better and finer person. The benefit may be the meaning the patient gives to the pain.

Pain to some people is viewed as punishment. Their suffering has been sent because of some past misdemeanours or inadequacies. They see themselves as those 'who for our evil deeds deserve to be punished', and are therefore receiving no more than what is justly due to them. It is rather unfortunate that the very word 'pain' comes into English from the French *peine*, derived through the Latin *poena* and ultimately from the Greek *poine* meaning 'penalty' or 'punishment'. Pain is therefore inflicted when one is 'bad', and it thereby comes as a signal for guilt. If it is deserved it seems all the more acceptable in spite of the discomfort.

Many patients suffering from cancer have feelings of guilt. Remorse for events in the past, broken relationships within the family, negligence in seeking medical aid, come to the forefront as they search for some sense of meaning in their predicament. In such circumstances both disease and pain are readily seen as punishment for 'sins' of commission and/or omission. Jacox and Stewart (1973) found that among a number of highly anxious patients with metastatic cancer there appeared a tendency to deny the existence of pain. This may relate to guilt feelings: 'I must have been wicked to have such pain as this.' Such thoughts lead readily to anger, bitterness and resentment: 'If this is what God does, so much for him.'

These negative emotional reactions prompt many a patient to find some way of atoning or undoing so that he may find relief by asking, 'Why me?' As he searches in vain for a satisfactory answer he undergoes a certain degree of confusion as to the meaning of his pain. There is a bitterness and resentment that others who are more wicked or sinful seem to get off 'scot free!' Resentment can readily progress to feelings of persecution and bedevilment.

Pain isolates, and often involves an 'aloneness', an 'apartness', a feeling of being cut off from others. Suffering excludes a person from normal everyday living. His 'world' has temporarily stopped, no longer is he actively involved in the 'trivial round' or 'the common task'. Work has been interrupted, engagements cancelled, hopes thwarted and perhaps ambition blunted. Pain alienates and we 'lose our place'.

Someone who was recovering from a severe car crash and had spent several weeks in hospital commented: 'If anybody had asked me my name then, I would have said, "My name is pain". I was nothing but pain – a throbbing being. Nobody can ever know what it is like.'

Pain separates a person from everyone else. Writing in severe pain from her hospital bed Cady (1976) comments:

The nurses avoid me. Is it because of my immature

107

behaviour during these periods of desperation? Is it because they feel frustrated by an inability to rid me of you (pain)? Oh, if only they knew how terribly lonely I feel when it's just the two of us together, and if only they knew how much their presence, their expressions of concern, and their mere touch do to strengthen me during these battles.

Patients are never so alone as when they are in severe pain. They are driven into themselves and become wholly occupied with their immediate concern which is the self. The childhood sorts of regression are often revived and they revert to being the centre of all concern. Every demand must be satisfied and every need supplied. 'In the loneliness of pain', observed LeShan (1964), 'only our existence is real. We float alone in space, conscious only of the suffering.' Feelings of isolation and abandonment intensify the pain experience. 'Loneliness', observed one patient, 'is not so much a matter of being alone as of not belonging. Everyone needs person-to-person contact.'

Feelings of loneliness in the pain of terminal illness bring a poignancy all of their own. They can lead to an excessive preoccupation with self, with an accompanying loss of interest in other people and things around. Ivan, in Tolstoy's *The Death of Ivan Ilych*, found 'a loneliness in the midst of a populous town and surrounded by numerous acquaintances and relations but that yet could not have been more complete anywhere – either at the bottom of the sea or under the earth – during that terrible loneliness Ivan Ilych had lived only in memories of the past'.

The attitudes of others in pain can influence our own reactions, particularly in the atmosphere of a hospital ward with a common sharing in a fellowship of suffering: 'It's something that happens to us all!'

There is, too, the 'pollyanna' attitude: the 'cheerful optimist' who makes the best of his own condition, and thinks of others who are in a far worse situation than himself.

Someone who himself had spent a long period in hospital and undergone a number of operations was sitting alongside the bed of a fellow-sufferer who suddenly exclaimed in a quiet voice:

Do you know, three times during the past week the pain

has been so bad that I have determined to end my own life rather than go on with it all, and each time just as I had made up my mind that suicide was the only way out I have thought of that poor devil upstairs and what he was going through, and I have said to myself, 'If he can stick what he has got and be cheerful, well so can you', and I have stayed my hand. (Childs, 1949)

There are patients who seem to regard their pain experience as their 'cross': 'This is my cross and I just have to grin and bear it.' 'He only puts it on those who are strong enough to bea⸱ it. If the cross was good enough for Christ it's good enough for me!'

Pain is seen as a means of identifying with the sufferings of Christ. God has some purpose for 'sending' the pain. When pain is thus seen as a deserved punishment it is often used to relieve guilt feelings and so endured with patience and tranquillity. Suffering and pain are looked upon as an effect of God's chastising love, and it is reckoned that if borne courageously without seeking relief spiritual benefits will accrue. 'I don't need to go to church, I'm doing my bit by taking all this pain upon myself,' remarked one patient who rigidly refused all analgesics.

To submit too readily to pain and suffering may be a sign of a craving for pity and the attention and affection of others: 'Look at what I am having to put up with.' Pain becomes glorified and idealised, a 'martyr syndrome', and is seen as in itself bestowing some special grace and sanctification.

The prostitute in the musical *Godspell* (Stephen Schwartz, 1972) sings that she will put a pebble in her shoe as a dare and follow Jesus: 'I shall call the pebble dare . . . dare shall be carried and when we both have had enough, I shall take him from my shoe singing, "We shall join you Lord and I'll take your hand finally glad".' The pain of such discomfort was to serve as a 'thorn in the flesh' to remind her she is striving to improve her way of life.

ATTITUDE OF THE CHILD

In a survey carried out by Schultz (1971) of the attitudes and perception of pain of ten and eleven-year-old children, it was found that the fear of death is one aspect of the perception of pain that this age-group experiences. In answer to the question, 'What does pain mean to you?', some of the replies were: 'It hurts, it hurts inside'; 'I feel like screaming'; 'I think I'm going to die'; 'Getting injections': 'It hurts so much it kills ya.' A similar survey carried out by the author resulted in identical responses:

I havent had too much pain in my time but I know it hurts (a lot). (N.C. aged 12)

A pain is a fing that hurts. (S. aged 9)

When I am in pain I feel sad. You don't know what to do. You get bored, angry, all worked up. Then start to feel sorry for yourself. (S. aged 11)

Pain is very sore and it can make you feel sad. Makes you cry – feel down in the dumps, and you don't like telling anybody about it. Some people can take the pain and some people can't. (P. aged 11)

I was scared. I thought I was going to die early. (G. aged 11)

Boys in middle childhood are expected to be strong, assertive and courageous. They are inclined to adopt a brave 'front', for 'only babies cry', 'big boys don't cry'. Girls, on the other hand, are allowed greater freedom to express their hurt feelings, their fears and emotional upsets. There is also a tendency among this particular age-group to be angry at themselves for being ill, and this often results in destructive, hostile and belligerent outbursts.

A common concept among young children is that pain is seen as punishment for some misdeed. Perhaps the patient has often been reprimanded at home and sent to bed or confined to his room for being naughty. Anna Freud (1952) states:

So far as his own interpretation is concerned the child in pain is a child maltreated, harmed, punished, persecuted, threatened by annihilation. The 'tough child' does not mind pain, not because he feels less or is more courageous in the real sense of the word, but because in his case latent

110

unconscious fantasies are less dominant and therefore less apt to be connected with the pain. Where anxiety derived from fantasy plays a minor or no part, even severe pain is borne well and quickly forgotten. Pain augmented by anxiety on the other hand, even if slight in itself, represents a major event in the child's life and is remembered a long time afterwards.

It is interesting to note that some eleven-year-old children view pain from a psychological point of view (in terms of tension, fear, loneliness, anxiety), revealing the beginning of the development of mature levels of thinking, whereas the majority of ten-year-olds discuss their pain in physical terms ('I feel sick in the stomach'). Savedra et al. (1982), in their study to determine how children describe the experience of pain, questioned a sample of 100 children in hospitals, and 114 children in church and private schools, all between nine and twelve years old. In reply to the question, 'What is good about pain?' 48 per cent said 'nothing' and 16 per cent, 'I don't know'. A twelve-year-old girl answered, 'It tells you something is wrong', and an eleven-year-old girl: 'It makes you experience things'. One nine-year-old girl in hospital responded: 'If there was no pain you wouldn't know like your hand was burning or not.' Only one child stated that pain was punishment.

As children have a limited verbal ability to describe their pain their drawings can be a helpful method to detect some of their attitudes. Unruh et al. (1983), in their study of children's drawings, observed that directly following surgery, red and black were reported as the colour of their pain. As the child began to recover and pain decreased, blue, yellow and eventually white were the colours most often associated with it. Pain was represented as an object which inflicts pain, or as a personality which is capable of causing pain. The children (five to eighteen years) most frequently portrayed themselves doing something to help cope with their pain, and the most common actions were the use of pressure, quiet and sleep.

Children always seem ready to express themselves if those around them are prepared to listen. The attentive presence of a caring and sensitive person allows a child to give vent to his feelings when in pain. He is somehow granted permission

111

to feel pain, and such outward and expressive feelings reduce his fear and anxiety.

There is great need for those who care for the child to work through their own anxiety and feelings of distress before they can effectively be of help and provide therapeutic support for children in pain and discomfort. Feelings of guilt can arise when medical and nursing staff may have to carry out procedures which they know will prove painful and probably add to the child's distress (see p. 97). In order to cope they either have to adopt a cold professional and clinical detachment, and repress subjective feelings and impulses, or care for him as a human being and look at the total, ever-changing attitudes of the child in relation to his pain. They first have to understand and appreciate how he perceives pain, take measures either to prevent or lessen it, and then proceed to help him as a partner rather than a victim.

GENERAL ATTITUDES

Illich (1975) emphasises the important moral function of pain. He sees pain as having a healing power, which prompts the sufferer to ask questions concerning not only the quality of his personal life but also the ultimate meaning of life in general. It is his belief that:

> medical civilisation . . . tends to turn pain into a technical matter and thereby deprives suffering of its inherent personal meaning. People unlearn the acceptance of suffering as an inevitable part of their conscious coping with reality and learn to interpret every ache as an indicator of their need for padding or pampering.

Much depends upon our readiness to accept the challenge of pain. Acceptance is no resigned passivity. It is rather to have the courage to face the facts, and to attempt to 'get inside' the pain and suffering. It is something far more profound than merely resigning ourselves to the inevitable, or submitting to a divine fiat. Bloom (1971) makes clear the distinction between resignation and surrender in the following terms:

> Resignation means to 'sign off', to resign from a function.

Surrender means such an act of trust and confidence that you can put yourself unreservedly, joyfully, by an act of freedom, into the hand of God, whatever happens, because you are sure of him, more than you are sure of anything else . . . 'No one is taking my life from me, I give it freely.' This is surrender, not resignation.

Acceptance diminishes guilt and grief and so lessens pain and suffering. There can be a redeeming quality in the very act of acceptance which is not only beneficial to the patient concerned but also an example for others. A fellowship of suffering is evident in many a hospital ward. In such a therapeutic environment the loneliness of pain is overcome and suffering is seen no longer as 'an individual problem which isolates but a human problem which calls forth love' (Degenaar, 1979). Pain is then able to be articulated in a significant way within a context of shared values, and so given value and meaning.

Modern society seems to have little sense of the nature and purpose of pain and regards it:

> as an unpleasant fact which, like every other evil, [it] must do [its] best to get rid of. To do this, it is generally held, there is no need for any reflection of the phenomenon itself . . . modern man is irritated by things which older generations accepted with equanimity. He is irritated by old age, long illness, and even by death; above all he is irritated by pain.

Buytendjik (1962) sees the consequences of this as 'an immoderate state of algophobia (fear of pain) which is itself an evil and sets a seal of timidity on the whole of human life'.

An intelligence test set for sixth-formers by the Saxon Ministry for Education to select candidates for the university, posed the question: 'Assume the discovery of a medicament freeing everyone to whom it is administered from all physical pains for the rest of his life. What would happen as the result of such an innovation?' Some of the sixth-formers thought it would be a very good idea as a most welcome remedy, although the reasons they advanced were often rather strange; for example: 'Doctors wouldn't have so much to do . . .' 'Doctors would become rather superfluous . . .' ' . . . Would

113

only be needed for setting broken bones . . .' 'Hospitals would be emptied . . .' A few asserted: 'You wouldn't get stomach ache no matter how much you ate'; 'You wouldn't get head-ache poring over difficult work, in short it would be wonderful.' There was no indication offered as to the positive significance of pain. There were some however who did suppose pain had some meaning. For example, one examinee stated: 'People would be even worse in consequence than they are now. They could afford every possible indulgence without disagreeable consequences. Their spiritual welfare would hardly trouble them . . . it would lead to selfishness, uniformity and utter indifference . . .' This final answer was the only one which arrived at a positive interpretation of pain, linking it with the whole purpose of life (Sauerbruch and Wenke, 1963).

Pain forces man to reflect, and it will be his inner attitude which will often help shape his ability to cope with his pain' experience and cultivate a powerful formative and trans-formative effect. Many patients bear their pain and discomfort with great courage and fortitude. It is not suffering per se which ennobles or enriches but the manner in which it is borne. Pain can never be neutral; it impels a human being to make a personal decision, an act of will. He must take some attitude towards it, for pain demands a personal answer from the individual. As the common companion of birth and growth, disease and death, it is 'a phenomenon deeply inter-twined with the very question of human experiences, and it often precipitates questioning the meaning of life itself' (Bakan 1968).

Bakan, D.   *Disease, Pain & Sacrifice: towards a psychology of suffering*. Beacon, Boston 1968.
Bloom, A.   'The theology of suffering', in *From Fear to Faith*, ed. N. Autton. SPCK, London 1971.
Buytendjik, F. J. J. *Pain: its modes and functions*. Univ. Chicago Press 1962.
Cady, J. W.   'Dear pain', *Amer. J. Nursing* (June 1976), pp. 950–1.

Childs, G. E. *A Parson's Thoughts on Pain*. Mowbray, London 1949.

Copp, L. A. 'The spectrum of suffering', *Amer. J. Nursing*, 74:3 (1974), pp. 491–5.
(ed.) *Recent Advances in Nursing: perspectives on pain*. Churchill Livingstone, Edinburgh 1985.

Davitz, L. J. and J. R. 'How do nurses feel when patients suffer?', *Amer. J. Nursing*, 75 (1975), pp. 1505–10.

Davitz, L. J., and Pendleton, S. 'Nurses' inferences of patient suffering', *Nurs. Res.*, 18 (1969), pp. 100–7.

Degenaar, J. J. 'Some philosophical considerations of pain', *Pain*, 7 (1979), pp. 281–304.

Diers, D., et al. 'Effect of nursing interaction on patients in pain', *Nursing Research*, 21 (1972), pp. 419–24.

Freud, A. 'The role of bodily illness in the mental life of children', in *The Psychoanalytical Study of the Child*, VII (1952), pp. 69–82.

Hayward, J. *Information: a prescription against pain; the study of nursing care*, Research Project, ser. 2, No. 5. RCN, London 1975.
'Pain: psychological and social aspects', *Nursing*, 1 (1980), pp. 21–7.

Illich, I. *Medical Nemesis: the exploration of health*. Calder & Boyars, London 1975.

Jacox, A. K. (ed.) *Pain: a source book for nurses and other health professionals*. Little, Brown, Boston 1977.

Jacox, A. K., and Stewart, M. 'Relations of psychosocial factors and type of pain', Paper presented at 9th Ann. Research Conf., San Antonio, Texas (21 March 1973), 5.

LeShan, L. 'The world of the patient in severe pain of long duration', *J. Chron. Dis.*, 17 (1964), pp. 119–26.

Lewis, C. S. *The Problem of Pain*. Fontana, London 1940.

Maguire, P. 'Consequence of poor communication between nurses and patients', *Nursing* (1985).
'Communication skills and patient care', in A. Steptoe and A. Matthews (eds), *Health*

	Care and Human Behaviour: Academic Press, London 1984.
Melzack, R., and Wall, P. D.	*The Challenge of Pain.* Penguin, London 1982.
Raiman, J.	'Pain relief: a two-way process', *Nursing Times* (9 April 1986), pp. 24–8.
Sauerbruch, F., and Wenke, H.	*Pain: its meaning and significance,* tr. E. Fitzgerald. Allen & Unwin, London 1963.
Savedra, M., et al.	'How do children describe pain? A tentative assessment', *Pain,* 14 (1982), pp. 95–104.
Schultz, N.	'How children perceive pain', *Nursing Outlook,* 19 (1971), p. 670.
Tolstoy, L.	*The Death of Ivan Ilych and Other Stories.* New American Library, 1960.
Unruh, A., et al.	'Children's drawings of their pain', *Pain,* 17 (1983), pp. 385–92.

6

Ministering to those in Pain

When pain is to be borne, a little courage helps more than much knowledge, a little human sympathy more than much courage, and the least tincture of the love of God more than all.

C. S. Lewis (1940)

Make me pain as you were once
made pain for me
that I may be for them what you have been
for them and me.

Ralph Wright (1977)

It is only those who have examined their own emotional needs and dealt with their own thoughts and philosophies of pain and suffering who are the better able to minister to patients struggling through doubt and fear with their present predicament. Those who minister have to look at themselves, their own thoughts and feelings, the manner in which they react in the presence of pain and suffering. They have to come to terms with their own spiritual distress when confronted with another's pain; their own emotional strengths and weaknesses have to be explored and understood if they are to exercise an enabling and supportive ministry. They will be blind to others' needs if their own anxiety and insecurity are too intense when faced with ontological questions. If they are in discomfort in the situation, carers will have the tendency to distance themselves from the sufferer. They must be able to feel with and yet be detached from the patient's emotions and anxieties if they are to be really sensitive to the other's wants and at the same time free to help. Patients in pain are apt to unmask the emotional and spiritual inadequacies of those striving to minister to them.

The pain and weariness we see in others are reminders of our own fragility and humanness. It may be that carers hasten to remove the pain and anguish of the patient because in identifying with him they cannot stand their own personal suffering and questioning. They have to learn to 'get themselves off their hands', and to understand and accept their own motivations; otherwise their endeavour to minister to those in pain, no matter how well intentioned, will soon be thwarted and unproductive.

RELATIONSHIPS

Every effort should be made, albeit often in a limited period, to try to understand and know the 'person' of the patient, his hopes and fears, his strengths and weaknesses, his joys and sorrows. The gift of discernment (cf. Phil. 1:9) affords an ability to grasp things as they really are; to acquire a discerning knowledge and understanding of human ills and the needs and conditions of those in crisis. Discernment means being alert to the loneliness, resentment and frustration behind the reported message: 'The doctor came and said . . . and did . . .' It involves a sensitive understanding of the awareness and discovery of the person behind the pain, helping him to feel at ease, to be himself. One patient in severe pain complained: 'You have not understood, because you do not know. I asked you one day how you would feel if, for eight whole days, you had never slept. You replied that such a thing never happened but that if it did, it would certainly not be pleasant. It is evident you do not understand' (Lériche, 1939). A person in pain is helped the moment he senses that he is beginning to be understood. A dying person was asked what he looked for above all in the people who were ministering to him. 'For someone to look as if they are trying to understand me,' he remarked. 'He did not look for success but only that someone should care enough to try' (Saunders, 1965).

The art of ministering centres on relationships – carer, patient, family, staff – which are based on confidence and trust. The integrity of relationship will prove far more important than any form of technique. It will involve a dialogue, an offering of ourself to another, the giving of ourself to another from the depths of our consciousness. Such communication will take place in both verbal and non-verbal contexts. 'Communication' is based on the Latin word *communis*, 'common'. When we communicate we are trying to establish a 'commonness' with someone. The first and most important premise is that words work within the context of certain feelings, and the helpfulness or otherwise of ministry will depend upon feelings rather than words. It involves staying with the patient in the frame of reference of his pain and suffering in a warm subject-to-subject or person-to-person relationship. The only instrument the carer has is himself, and his approach has to be receptive, open and warm. Much that will be said verbally will often be emphasised non-verbally. Non-verbal clues have to be observed for many patients communicate through their pain, especially the inarticulate and inhibited personalities.

Communication involves so much more than words. 'Body-language' can contribute to the total expression of feeling and mood. A patient in pain notices the expression on the face of the carer and relates it to his own needs and anxieties. He will validate his self-feelings by what he hears in the voice and sees in the eyes of those about him. Direct eye-contact or mutual glance conveys a message of focused attention to the concerns of the sufferer, and such a sense of caring, relationship and companionship creates an atmosphere of openness or 'space' in which he is more ready to express what is in his heart, rather than what he thinks others want him to say. A good listener looks at the speaker, and facial expressions speak a universal language. 'I saw his heart in his face,' wrote Shakespeare (*The Winter's Tale*, Act 1, Scene 2). True relationship can only take place in the setting of genuine personal communication, in the sharing of person with person as a whole being with a whole being.

In an atmosphere of 'togetherness' and 'alongsidedness' the carer will allow both patient and family to give full vent to their feelings, and will not be threatened by the doubts which might be expressed, the anger, bitterness or despair. His function will be to extend a relationship, offer companionship, work through fears, struggle with doubts and share frustrations. The patient will be allowed to take the initiative in any discussion while the carer will offer support and counsel that are relevant to the patient's feelings and the gravity or otherwise of the situation, rather than give way to over-assurance, unnecessary circumlocutions and untruths. The patient will be helped to express what he wants to express, what he wants to say yet finds difficult to put into words. When patients make small talk in the presence of big problems it is usually not that they do not want to talk about important issues but that they do not know how. The carer has to learn the language by which others not only reveal themselves but also conceal themselves, so that his words not only help but heal.

Prolonged pain, continual discomfort, can induce feelings of despair, rejection and loss of will to live. Such moods are to be accepted and understood rather than made occasion for moralising or reasoning. Those who minister will watch with those in pain, relate to them, communicate with them, learn from them, without necessarily knowing all the answers. Such ministry symbolises our togetherness as a family, and such care and companionship often prove a kind of redemptive presence that becomes of itself a valuable aid to recovery. In crisis of pain people are faced with questions of the ultimate as well as of the immediate concern. There will be occasions when the 'doing' will need to give way to the 'being' and 'being with', to allow the carer to develop enough inner space in which a meaning communication can take place.

MINISTRY OF 'PRESENCE'

The most important aspect of ministering may be the simple act of sitting at the bedside of the patient in pain. Being present can often be the most effective tranquilliser of all, symbolising 'I care', and offering 'the therapeutic use of self'. When the patient is alone, isolated and unoccupied his pain can easily become the focus of his attention and monopolise his thoughts and feelings. Isolation appears to weaken the ability to deal with crisis, to cope with pain and to fight for life. When in pain one is alone with oneself. The supports of status, prestige, independence, diminish considerably. 'Pain is always something new for him who suffers but banal to those about him,' wrote Daudet (1934).

'Being with' indicates not only a physical presence but also a sense of being available and accessible to the patient. The carer stays confident that he is of help, that his presence has meaning for himself as well as the patient. It is often assumed, be the carer nurse, physician or priest, that there is some magical protection against personal reaction to pain and suffering, while at the same time endowing him with an exquisite sense of sensitivity and compassion. The real fact is that there is a great deal of mental, emotional and spiritual strain involved in ministering to those in pain. The carer is constantly being reminded of his own finiteness and limited capacity. The 'being' and 'being with' require a deep conviction of the worth of what he is doing and an awareness of the help he can bring (Benoliel and Crowley, 1973).

What really matters to those in pain is that there is someone who is prepared to stay so that 'presence' is shared. A faithful presence, a caring heart and a listening ear afford the sufferer an opportunity to 'borrow strength'. Copp (1985) illustrates how a presence creates labels for the coping process, assisted by those who are prepared 'to be there':

Witness: 'When I get home I won't be able to tell the family what the pain was like but he will.'
Strength-lender: 'Even if I have my eyes closed because the pain is so bad, I know she is there and that helps me hold on.'
Verbal monitor: The patient in pain copes by giving a carefully reported account of the frequency, duration and severity of the pain: 'Oh dear, it's coming again – this is the worst yet.'

The healing resource of companionship and mutual concern is reflected vividly in Psalm 23:4: 'Even though I walk through a valley dark as death I fear no evil, for thou art with me'. Leventhal and Everhart (1979) tell of a pregnant woman in labour who sent her husband away for several hours during which time her labour pain intensified tremendously only to decrease when he returned to stay with her. Being with

121

someone in pain helps to resolve the aloneness, the apartness, the feelings of isolation of the sufferer. The fresh peasant lad who was prepared to stay with Ivan, in *The Death of Ivan Ilych* (Tolstoy, 1960), brought him much comfort and support during his spasms of great pain. Tolstoy relates how Ivan liked talking to him: 'Health, strength, and vitality in other people were offensive to him, but Gerasim's strength and vitality did not mortify but soothed him.' It was only with him that Ivan felt at ease, 'and in Gerasim's attitude towards him there was something akin to what he wished for, and so that attitude comforted him'. Staying with the patient diminishes his feelings of loneliness and fear of abandonment: it means in one sense sharing in the pain. Real words of comfort can only come from within, and can only be endured on a basis of a true unity of being. Then we no longer speak of 'suffering' but of 'your suffering', which through 'creative presence' becomes 'my suffering'.

EMPATHY

In an ancient tale the wise man said to the king, '*I* am the most important person in your life – because you are talking to me *now*.'

It is important to give the patient that sense of the 'now', which is the only moment in which he can ever live. There are some patients who revive memories of yesterday's pain as well as anticipating tomorrow's. One expressed it rather graphically: 'I always lived as if there were only tomorrow and yesterday. Today didn't exist.'

He who ministers can only become involved in the very existence and predicament of those in pain, their tensions, sufferings, meanings and values, through a deeply empathetic experience. If he is only prepared to stand off at a distance because of the threat to his own vulnerability he will assume a relationship of control, manipulation or domination. He needs to seek to understand how patients feel by honestly admitting to himself how he would feel should he be in similar circumstances, and take seriously the meaning the patient attaches to his experience.

Someone once turned Pilate's question, '*Quid est veritas?*'

'What is truth?' into the anagram, '*Est vir qui adest*', 'It is the man before you'. To be aware fully of that individualised truth in love and compassion is the substance of empathy. Buber (1937) in his concept of the 'I-Thou' emphasises the world of relation: 'The aim of relation is relation's own being, that is, contact with the "thou".' He prefers the term 'inclusion' rather than empathy; the 'inclusion' of the other person which involves a 'living through' of a common event from the standpoint of the other – a shared experience. Reik (1948) makes reference to the empathetic process of 'listening with the third ear', which denotes an instinctive capacity of the unconscious to 'hear' the unspoken communications of another. Rogers (1962) defines such a warm creative relationship as sensing 'the client's private world as if it were your own, but without ever losing the "as if" quality – this is empathy'. It is a sincere and genuine effort to understand the unique fears and feelings of those in pain. Rogers stresses the importance of the patient's perceiving that someone is trying to understand his meaning.

A graphic portrayal of the healing effect of such a relationship is given by Morris West (1981) in his great novel, *The Clowns of God*. Jean Marie, the exiled Pope, is visiting his friend Carl Mendelius who lies desperately ill in hospital after the explosion of a letter-bomb.

> 'Carl, this is Jean. Can you hear me?' There was an answering pressure against his palm and more helpless gurgling as Mendelius tried in vain to articulate. 'Please don't try to talk. We don't need words, you and I. Just lie quiet and hold my hand. I will pray for both of us.' He said no words. He made no ritual gestures. He simply sat by the bed, clasping Mendelius' hand between his own, so that it was as if they were one organism: the whole and the maimed, the blind and the seeing man. He closed his eyes, and opened his mind, a vessel ready for the inpouring of the Spirit, a channel by which it might infuse itself into the conjoined consciousness of Carl Mendelius.

The result of that pastoral visit was that 'there was a calm so powerful that he could feel the fevered pulse of the sick man subside like sea waves after a storm'.

There can be no empathy where there is authoritarianism.

123

Stereotyped and rigid attitudes make those in pain feel dependent and inferior and deprived of personal decision-making, and openness of feelings. 'If a person stays with me . . . and he will be able to help . . . when anyone comes to visit me, I don't want him to come with his own agenda,' pleads JoAnn Kelley Smith (1977), during the pain of her terminal illness.

'Agenda anxiety' speaks of the insecurity of the carer who to his own satisfaction feels compelled to get across all the points, and cover all the subjects. Such compulsive talking can be a means of avoiding what others are trying to say. Too frequent questioning implies standing opposite rather than beside the patient, and so directing and controlling the conversation. 'He who asks the questions', states Balint (1964), 'will get answers, but not much else.' A person in crisis needs 'you' not your answers. 'Why do you keep what we need most from us,' remarked one patient. 'Don't you know that if you don't give us something of yourself as a person you can't mean anything to us at all!'

Empathy has to be seen in contrast to sympathy. Sympathy is the act or capacity of entering into or sharing the feelings of another. Empathy is a 'feeling into' and is dependent to a great extent on the richness of our own experience; it has to do with the matured use of the self. Aring (1958) describes the process as;

> not only an identification of souls, but unlike the implication of sympathy it is an awareness of one's separatedness from the observed. One has had one's own feelings and relationships, and has worked at the understanding of them, and they will be useful in understanding those feelings and relationships of others.

A doctor who for many years has been suffering bouts of severe acute pain, which he describes as 'knife-thrusts' and 'vice-like grips', states that;

> the one thing I am quite sure those of us who live with pain do not want is sympathy in the way so many people think of it. We do not want people constantly telling us that they are sorry for us. All we do ask is that people understand that living with pain makes demands on us,

and that if occasionally we do not feel quite ourselves, that is understandable.

Our ability to exercise an empathetic care of pain sufferers depends greatly on the richness of our own emotional experiences, the ability to understand our own feelings and relationships, and by reason thereof, those of others. There is no knowing so useful in our ministry as the knowledge of ourselves.

LISTENING

Silence can be the most effective instrument of communication. To listen is often the most effective way for the carer to 'talk' to those in pain, and to communicate the attitudes which are so important. The counsellor will listen skilfully, sensitively, sympathetically for clues which indicate either a readiness to discuss or a wish to remain silent. The patient must be given 'space' to think and to feel, as well as 'permission' to express both thoughts and feelings openly and honestly. Empathetic listening identifies with the patient's pain problems, hopes and aspirations, and whatever anguish is being expressed. There is always the ever-present temptation, which must be resisted, to look for answers instead of listening to questions. The skilled listener will interpret shades of meaning expressed verbally or non-verbally, the significance of gestures and the implication of responses. He will listen with heart and eyes as well as ears and soon discover that those in pain communicate all kinds of attitudes and emotional reactions by their very gestures. What is the patient 'saying' with his body, his facial expression, his movements? What area of pain or discomfort is he trying to communicate?

By his listening and by his capacity to read and interpret the complete language of those in pain, he will enable the patient to answer for himself so much that he has sought from others. The carer will listen to the 'spaces' between the words expressed, and search for the implications of the pain for each unique individual. Commenting on the nature of such true human sincerity, true transparency, Tournier (1957) describes it as a rare and difficult thing, and emphasises how much depends upon the person who is listening. He writes:

There are those who pull down the barriers and make the way smooth; there are those who force the doors and enter our territory like invaders; there are those who barricade us, shut us in upon ourselves, dig ditches and throw walls around us; there are those for whom we always remain strangers, speaking an unknown tongue. And when it is our turn to listen, which of these are we for? That should make us think of God, who is not only *one* who says: 'Listen to me', but also *one* who says: 'I am listening to you'.

The middle-aged patient who explained that her pain 'seems to be tearing me apart' was yearning for security and meaning, and spoke not only of her physical needs but of the complex interaction of her emotional, social and spiritual problems. The emotional facets of those in pain, fear of the unknown, depression, anxiety, are the more able to be identified by means of a listening ministry, and by a mutual sharing and working through together, for fantasy and imagination play major roles in the context of crisis.

PHYSICAL TOUCH

Physical touch symbolises a sensitive communication in empathetic relationships. The gesture conveys a message, one of caring and concern. It has been suggested by Rubin (1963) that in situations of intense personal stress in which the patient feels vulnerable and isolated no other modality of communication can be compared in immediacy to the comforting and quieting effects of touch. Physical touch decreases the level of anxiety and reinforces a component of security and warmth. It is an act which symbolises understanding, comfort and interest, and may often lead on to verbal interchange. A patient recalling her husband's presence and support at her bedside during a prolonged and painful illness remarked: 'Often he didn't have to say a word, but merely held me, and the holding, touching and implicit concern were supportive enough' (Cady, 1976).

In discussing what methods other than drugs they had found therapeutic to alleviate pain, a number of nurses mentioned the importance of physical touch:

126

I have found simply talking with patients helps – understanding them and what they're going through. Often just being with them is therapeutic so that they know they're not alone – and touching them gently and soothingly; stroking their forehead or holding their hand. I have found it helpful to perform the bedbath with my hands rather than a flannel, i.e. washing the back is especially relaxing in certain cases. The importance of touch is quite extraordinary, I think – perhaps because it reduces some of the fear in the patient and therefore helps them to cope with the pain. (4th year nursing student)

A sympathetic attitude; touching, cuddling – that is, obvious affection and love so the patient, or person experiencing the pain, knows someone cares for the way they feel. Also simple physical attendance, such as wiping the patient's face, combing their hair, etc. can be a comfort. (1st year nursing student)

From my limited experience, just being with somebody and holding his hand can help a great deal. Sitting worrying alone makes illness and pain grow out of proportion in many cases. Having company, someone to talk to, does a world' of good to a patient's state of mind. Also keeping occupied to 'divert the mind' really helps. It is easy to dwell on misery and imagine being worse than is really the case, until a nurse, a friend, or relation renews the will and enthusiasm to get better. (1st year nursing student)

THE PATIENT'S NEEDS

Those in pain need *love*. They need to experience love far more than pity, a love which is experienced through human relationships. The carer can offer additional love to that already being given in many instances by families and friends, or a substitute love when other supporters are non-existent or unable to fulfil their supportive role because of personal unmet needs. Pain sufferers are particularly sensitive to feelings and moods, and in their vulnerability pity reinforces aggression and serves to weaken the striving to retain dignity. Lewis (1960) in writing of human love makes the distinction between 'need-love' and 'gift-love'. What those in pain need is not only the former, the attention for which they crave in their distress, but also the latter, that divine gift of love which enables the carer to give of his all and to love to the uttermost.

Hope, so essential to those in pain, is no static act or aspiration but is dynamic, full of thoughts, feelings and actions that change from time to time. 'It is a peculiarity of man', writes Frankl (1964), 'that he can only live by looking to the future – sub specie aeternitis.' The patient needs *concrete* hope – release from pain, the ability to achieve certain goals such as longer periods of relief, more freedom of movement – as well as *abstract* hope, the element of transcendence described by Emily Dickinson:

> 'Hope' is the thing with Feathers
> That perches in the soul
> And sings the tune without the words
> And never stops
> At all . . .

'I just go on hoping,' said a patient who was suffering long continued bouts of pain. Such *generalised* hope gives a positive aspect to present circumstances; it serves to counteract despair and restore the purpose of life. *Particularised* hope centres round a hope object – improvement and relief of pain, a sense of meaning in life, an incentive to co-operate. When hope is encouraged and supported by those who minister the patient feels strengthened and renewed, full of purpose and courage. All such positive expectations and hope for the future need to be stimulated.

Kubler-Ross's (1969) counsel not to deprive the dying patient of hope is also applicable to those living in pain. The patient has to be helped to have complete trust and confidence in members of the health team, the continuity of their care and the security of their companionship. In his anxiety to be of the maximum support the carer will need to beware of unfulfilled and rash promises of relief. There is the ever-present temptation to offer exaggerated hope. An important element of hope is in helping the patient to face the reality of his problems and his pain. Such hope gives life a sense of purpose and meaning.

Absence of hope obstructs the patient's achieving this fullness, meaning and purpose. Recounting his experience in the concentration camps Frankl (1964) relates how they had to teach the despairing men 'that it did not matter what we expected from life, but rather what life expected from us . . . any attempt to restore a man's inner strength in camp had first to succeed in showing him some future goal'. Those in pain and suffering need a future orientation, a challenge which motivates them to move out of their slough of despond and on to the ground of hope.

The skilled counsellor will not build castles of hope in the air; sincere hope cannot be built upon false expectations. Hope is not to be conveyed as sheer optimism or wishful thinking: it is not built upon naive and unrealistic ideals. Christian hope is entirely realistic and reckons with the worst: it goes to the heart of forgiveness and is closely allied with faith and trust. A profound depression, anger turned inwards, is possibly the most consistent result of hopelessness. Hope as a positive force seems to have been much neglected in the care of those in pain.

Another important need of the patient is that he is 'given permission' to express whatever anger and hostility he might feel and know that such sentiments will be met with support and understanding. He should feel safe and secure enough to be angry if necessary, rather than be urged to be an example of patience and piety to others. Far too many patients turn their anger inwards and experience guilt and depression. If anger is channelled aright it can become a positive and productive emotional reaction. Signs of anger can be evidenced in avoidance of eye-contact and vocal withdrawal. It is important to find out why the pain sufferer is angry, and assist him to give full vent to his feelings.

The carer may feel threatened when confronted by such anger on account of his own perception of anger, or a failure to appreciate its significance to the patient. He may feel uncomfortable in the face of strong negative emotion, but should attempt to help the patient in his anger to accept himself as feeling angry, and neither defend nor reject him but rather allow him to realise that it is safe for him to express his feelings freely and naturally. It is helpful to explore together the anger's etiology. A Jewish prayer states that to 'rail' is not necessarily to 'rebel'. If the patient were not angry he would probably be extremely depressed.

For a patient in acute pain a spirit of fortitude and a sense of security is often instilled by reassurance. However it is important that it should be properly timed, for when indiscriminately and blandly used it is likely to create problems, doubts and uncertainties, and become counter-productive. It needs to be utilised with more than platitude or in such banal expressions as, 'Don't worry, you'll be all right. Your pain will soon pass.' Reassurance discreetly used gives a sense of hope and confidence and an incentive for living. It can become an effective tool in reducing the patient's anxiety and foster concentration on recovery, as well as a readiness to bear what has to be borne, both of illness and of treatment.

Although in the psychotherapeutic setting reassurance is often frowned upon as a therapeutic procedure ('reassurance never reassures'), often motivated as it is by the therapist's own need for reassurance because of anxiety stirred up by a client in distress, yet reassuring information can often bring much relief to a patient in acute pain. One patient after surgery remarked: 'When I was told it was all removed I first wanted to know over and over again. Every time someone came I needed to know that I was going to be all right. Once isn't enough' (Small, 1977). Many a patient can bear acute pain if he knows it will not be prolonged and what the symptoms connote. Some find consolation in the knowledge that other people are suffering from a similar complaint to theirs. A rather humorous illustration is given by Robert Morley (1970):

> There is a lot to be said for the country surgery which I patronise ... Both partners employ a phrase in consultation of which I am particularly fond and which I always find immensely reassuring. Whether it is pink-eye, incipient tonsillitis, an ingrowing toenail, or high blood pressure from which I believe myself to be suffering, they allay my anxiety with a simple statement that there is a lot of it about. I find it so comforting to realise that most of the inhabitants of my village ... are currently fighting the same dread symptoms.

A patient in pain needs to be helped to create his own *personal meaning* and to integrate his suffering with his personal goals and values. Kahlil Gibran, in *The Prophet* (1926), reveals that 'your pain is the breaking of the shell that encloses your understanding'. Wherever possible the patient must be enabled to articulate his own meaning of pain, and to search for the answer which has most meaning for him, for it cannot be provided by other persons no matter how well intentioned and sincere. No one can create meaning for another, only enable or inhibit it. In terminal pain there exists the tension between 'hanging on' and 'letting go', which often creates a spiritual crisis, and affords an opportunity for growth.

Mount (1984) quotes the reaction of a cancer patient who reflects: 'It cut very deeply into me, but in cutting into me it opened me up . . . I'm changed; I'll always be changed. I'll always be happier for what I have gone through.' The carer can help those in pain ask questions and seek meaning, but at the same time be conscious of the fact that he will be unable to provide answers or solutions. What 'meaning' is for the patient is highly individual and unique. What can I bring out of this situation? What is my condition saying to me?

If pain and crisis are viewed as meaningless they may cause the patient to suffer spiritually, so the wise counsellor will offer him objectives for living, goals in life that are real to him. 'If there is a meaning in life at all, then there is a meaning in suffering. Suffering is an inevitable part of life, even as fate and death' (Frankl, 1964). Where there is no sense of life, no aim, no purpose, the will to live soon becomes paralysed. 'Suffering', wrote Spinoza, 'ceases to be suffering as soon as we form a clear and precise picture of it'. It is how the patient in pain is enabled to grow through the experience, rather than the experience itself, which is all important. In periods of pain there are often no answers, but what is far more important is to search for meaning. In self-exploration and self-acceptance there comes growth, and the patient is enabled to become a fuller and richer person, not defeated and beaten, but stronger and more complete.

THE FAMILY'S NEEDS

The patient should not be seen in isolation from his family, for the needs of family and patient are inseparable. It was a middle-aged patient who remarked: 'We are a very closely-knit family, and when one of us is sick we're all pretty sick.' A constructive approach in the care of those in pain must therefore take account of the family as a whole. How is the family reacting? Do they understand the illness? Do they always have to be doing something? Have they already given up hope, and so convey grief rather than empathy? What are some of their emotional and spiritual strengths and weaknesses? The attitudes of the family are of vital importance, and in influencing its members the carer will be serving the patient. Attitudes and emotional states are contagious, especially in times of anxiety and regression. The family members have to be enabled to face up to their real fears and doubts; to look at themselves and be honest and open.

The cry of helplessness of those near and dear to patients in pain will often be heard: 'It is a terrible thing, a thing that we must all at some time have suffered, that feeling that someone you love is suffering and you can do nothing to help,' writes Gerald Vann (1947). He goes on to explain that there are two sorts of activity. There is the outgoing activity: the healing work of the hands, the comforting word, the little service that can bring consolation; and sometimes these are impossible. He suggests, however, that another sort of activity is purely inward; and this he sees as always possible and always healing. It is the activity of thought and love:

> You may have to say there is nothing I can do, nothing of outward activity . . . [but] you need never say, purely and simply, 'There is nothing I can do' . . . There are times when outward business only makes matters worse, *when, though it may bring you yourself relief,* it must be for the other at worst an additional exacerbation of suffering.

When a person is facing pain and discomfort with a new image of himself as weakened and dependent, his family relationships are likely to be troubled by his own subjective attitudes. Twycross (1975) shows how reactions can vary and are difficult to predict, for 'the small, physically frail woman may be a tower of strength, while the tough "he-man" finds himself unable to cope'. Physical pain can often give rise to the expression of strong emotions and conflicts. The experience of illness which disrupts the normal everyday life of the family may often bring to the surface not only the intense feelings being borne in present circumstances, but also other negative emotions which have been hidden and suppressed within the lower consciousness over a long period. Where such strong negative feelings exist they will need to be 'drained off', rather than be met with ready-made 'Christian answers'.

Implicit in the experience of pain lurks the threat of 'non-being' and this brings to light the whole area of religious concepts and values. The chronic pain sufferer may pine and grieve for the past; he may 'mourn' his loss and deprivation. His family too grieve for him and because of him. Questions of 'ultimate concern' loom large on the horizon, and a religious crisis can be precipitated in both family and patient by the circumstances of sickness and pain. Why did this have to happen to *us?* The deeper beliefs of the family are put to the test and it is important that ministry is concerned with the ongoing web of the patient's interpersonal relationships and the *total* situation taken into account. Families in existential situations of crisis are to be helped to find their way through to a sense of meaning and a creative issue 'out of all their afflictions'.

The challenge of the carer is to strengthen the resolve of the family, to understand and help clarify conflict, to initiate new patterns of adjustment, to deepen the sense of religious reality, and so represent through presence and empathy a genuine love and concern.

MINISTRY OF 'ABSENCE'

Physical closeness may in some instances increase a sense of pain. There are patients who just wish to be alone and their feelings are to be respected. Very few of those suffering from the pain of a migraine, for example, would want people to remain at their bedside. Other patients who value self-control may not feel free to give full vent to their feelings, shout, cry, or 'lose control', in the presence of another. As well as an art of 'arriving' and 'being with', there is also an art of 'creative withdrawal', the ability to be articulately absent. In our withdrawing we can help create 'space' for the Holy Spirit to be operative and in which by our absence God can become 'more present'.

'It is for your own good that I am going because unless I go, the Advocate will not come to you' (John 16:7). Not only does this thought make the minister sensitive to the last words which he speaks on leaving the patient, states Nouwen (1982), but it also puts the possibility of a prayer into a new perspective. In our endeavour to minister to the needs of those in pain there can be 'too much presence and too little absence, too much staying . . . and too little leaving them, too much of us and too little of God and his Spirit'. In our adherence to such a 'ministry of absence' our illusions of personal indispensability soon become unmasked.

PASTORAL CARE

Spiritual help needs to be exercised with the utmost tact and sensitivity. It becomes so glib to offer sermonettes about the benefits of pain, or murmur consoling words with 'silver-lining' approaches.

> We are so clumsy with the pain
> of other people
> we – so full of comfort so content
> to toss our velvet
> coated words
> like crusts to beggars – fail to diagnose
> the nausea men feel for trite maxims.'
> (Ralph Wright, 1977)

Those who minister have to try to understand how the patient is feeling; they will help him see pain as an accepted part of life rather than the belief that he has become a hapless victim to a senseless fate or of a blind chance. If the sufferer is able to conceive of his pain in this way his powers to resist it and bear it are being strengthened. Where prayer, the laying on of hands, and sacrament are used sensitively and selectively much spiritual strength and inner peace of mind may be derived through intimacy with God and the presence of another. Those who are at peace within themselves seem better able to bear their pain than those who are bitter and resentful. The healing of attitudes becomes therefore an essential part of ministry.

Saunders (1967), Kubler-Ross (1969), Lammerton (1973) and Hinton (1974) all emphasise how the presence of a person who is loved, trusted, and respected, and in whom the sufferer has full confidence, can have a significant impact on the intensity of his pain. Such compassionate attention counteracts the loneliness and helps to convey hope, love and understanding.

Essex (1984), writing during her painful terminal illness, recorded that she had:

> always supposed, that, in times of pain, one would automatically and naturally turn to one's prayers to gain comfort and help. But I found in fact that praying in pain was well nigh impossible. A black cloud of pain overshadowed almost everything else. I found that I had lost the power of concentration. The words of the lovely and familiar prayers I had been accustomed to use seemed to float away from me. 'Just rest in the presence of the Lord,' I said to myself. But I found that the realisation of the Lord's presence was difficult to grasp.

There may be many patients in pain who have feelings of frustration and guilt on account of their inability to pray. They become despondent at their apparent loss of faith and their failure to sustain their own personal religious standards or those set by their family or local church. They can be shown that often the desire or intention itself, an act of will, will become the prayer. So many sufferers in pain have to depend wholly upon the prayers of the carers and upon those of the whole Church. The prayers of the chaplain are to be coupled with those of all who minister in their respective spheres, the physicians, nurses, social workers, the great family of carers. 'You realise then', remarked a patient who was suffering a long progressively painful disease, 'what it is to belong to a family – there's a one-ness: you are being "borne up", and you derive great strength as a consequence.'

Pain is something that can be shared with the whole of the

Christian family. 'If you belong to a caring congregation, as I do,' recalled Essex, 'you know that the other members are praying for you and with you, and that through the very darkest attacks of pain the christian family is carrying you on a kind of cushion of prayer, making up what you cannot help but lack.' Prayer helps the patient to a realisation of the presence of Christ within, and can lead through pain to peace and tranquillity.

MINISTRY

In all our endeavours to minister we have to take the risk of being hurt, of being 'wounded' in the process, as we struggle to take the pain and brokenness of the other into our consciousness. It is in this way we all become 'wounded healers', following in the footsteps of our Lord himself. In the play, *The Angel that Troubled the Waters*, by Thornton Wilder, the apparently whole physician is commanded to stand back at the crucial moment, despite his own yearning for wholeness. 'Without your wound where would your power be?' asks the Angel. 'In love's service only the wounded soldiers can serve. Draw back.'

Only by accepting our own limitations and acknowledging our own wounds shall we be enabled to go beyond them. There will be many occasions when we shall have to say in utter honesty and sincerity, 'I don't know. I don't understand.' We can only be aware of pain and suffering which are our own. We can sympathise and try to enter into the experience of the other but the real feelings of those in pain will always be to us a closed book. When we try to explore the inner world of the patient we may be able to say, 'I know what pain is like,' but we cannot truthfully say: 'I know what *your* pain is like.' No one can fully share in the anguish of another.

Often we shall feel utterly inadequate but there is much consolation to be gained from some words of Saunders and Baines (1983), who remind us that 'the command – "Watch with me" – did not mean "Take this crisis away": it could not have meant "Explain it"; the simple, yet costly demand was "Stay there and stay awake".' Those who are prepared to do just that will find themselves trusting in a presence that can more easily reach the patient and his family, and endeavouring to use all their competence with love, sincerity, and compassion. If we cannot share in the pain of the other we can at least share with the other part of ourselves.

There may be little of the dramatic or the sensational, still less of the miraculous, in our ministry to those in pain, yet we shall be privileged to glimpse more than a little of the strength, the courage, the dignity of our fellow-men and become aware that the way each accepts his predicament is the measure of his human fulfilment. Pain is far more than something to be abolished, and if by our love, concern and care we help those who suffer to see their pain in terms of meaning and significance, then, as Degenaar (1979) states, their whole experience passes beyond the original Latin *poena*, 'punishment', to the Sanskrit root *pu* – purification.

Aring, C. D.	'Sympathy and empathy', J. Amer. Med. Ass., 167:4 (1958) pp. 448–52.
Balint, M.	'The doctor's therapeutic function', *Lancet*, 1 (1964), pp. 1177–80.
Benoliel, J. Q., and Crowley, D. M.	'The patient in pain: new concepts' *Proceedings of National Conf. on Cancer Nursing.* Univ. Washington, Seattle (10 September 1973).
Buber, M.	*I and Thou*. Scribners, New York 1937.
Cady, J. W.	'Dear pain', *Amer. J. Nurs.*, 76:6 (1976), pp. 960–1.
Copp, L. A.	'The spectrum of suffering', *Amer. J. Nurs.*,74 (1974), pp. 491–5, (ed.) *Recent Advances in Nursing: perspectives on pain*. Churchill Livingstone, Edinburgh 1985.
Daudet, A.	Qu. in N. Autton, *Pastoral Care in Hospitals*. SPCK (1968), p. 27
Degenaar, J. J.	'Some philosophical considerations on pain', *Pain*, 7 (1979), pp. 281–304.
Essex, R.	'Prayer in the midst of pain', *Church Times* (16 November 1984).

Frankl, V. E.   *Man's Search for Meaning*. Hodder &
                       Stoughton, London 1964.
Gibran, K.   *The Prophet*. Heinemann, London 1926.
Hinton, J.   *Dying*, 2nd edn (Penguin, London 1972),
                       p. 159.
                       'Talking with people about to die', *BMJ*, 3
                       (1974), pp. 25–7.
Kubler-Ross, E.   *On Death and Dying*. Macmillan, New York
                       1969.
Lammerton, R.   *Care of the Dying*. Priory Press, 1973.
Lériche, R.   *The Surgery of Pain*. Baillière, Tindall & Cox,
                       London 1939.
Leventhal, H. and   'Emotion, pain and physical illness', in
   Everhart, D.   *Emotions in Personality and Psychopathology*, ed.
                       C. E. Izard. Plenum Press, New York 1979.
Lewis, C. S.   *The Four Loves*. Bles, London 1960.
Morley, R.   *World Med.* (25 November 1970), qu. in N.
                       Kessel, 'Doctor and patient: reassurance',
                       Lancet (26 May 1979), pp. 1128–33.
Mount, B. M.   'Psychological and social aspects of cancer
                       pain', in *Textbook of Pain*, ed. P. D. Wall and
                       R. Melzack. Churchill Livingstone,
                       Edinburgh 1984.
Nouwen, H. J. M.   *The Living Reminder*. Gill & Macmillan,
                       1982.
Reik, T.   *Listening with the Third Ear*. Grove Press,
                       New York 1948.
Rogers, C.   'The interpersonal relationship: the core of
                       guidance', *Harvard Educ. Review*, 32 (1962)
                       pp. 416–29.
Rubin, R.   'Maternal touch', *Nurs. Outlook*, 11 (1963),
                       pp. 828–31.
Saunders, C.   'Watch with me,' *Nursing Times* (26
                       November 1965).
                       The Management of Terminal Illness. Hosp.
                       Med. Publ., London 1967.
Saunders, C., and   *Living with Dying: the management of terminal
   Baines, M.   disease*. OUP, 1983.
Small, K.   'Elective Dissertation,' Manchester Univ.
                       Med. School (1977), qu. in N. Kessel,
                       'Doctor and patient: reassurance', *Lancet* (26
                       May 1979), pp. 1128–33.

Smith, J. K.   *Free Fall*. SPCK, London 1977.

Tolstoy, L.   *The Death of Ivan Ilych*. New American
                        Library, 1960.

Tournier, P.   *The Meaning of Persons*. SCM, London
                        (1957), p. 165.

Twycross, R. G.   *The Dying Patient*. Christian Med.
                        Fellowship, 1975.
                        A Time to Die, Christian Med. Fellowship,
                        1984.

Vann, G.   *The Pain of Christ and the Sorrow of God*,
                        Blackfriars, London 1947.

West, M.   *The Clowns of God* (Hodder & Stoughton,
                        London 1981), pp. 217–18.

Wright, R.   *Ripples of Stillness*. St Paul Editions, 1977.

Index of Names

Anderson, J. E. 71
Apley, J. 85
Aring, C. D. 124
Aristotle 3
Aquinas 16

Baines, M. 46, 136
Bakan, D. 114
Balint, M. 61, 124
Barnes, E. 19
Baskerville, P. A. 34
Becker, R. D. 81
Beecher, H. K. 14
Benoliel, J. Q. 38, 121
Benson, H. 52
Berne, E. 36
Beyer, J. E. 71
Bloom, A. 112
Bond, M. R. 39
Bonica, J. J. 6, 28, 32
Boom, C. ten 47
Bowlby, J. 73, 76, 77
Bradley, N. C. A. 61
Browning, R. 48
Bruegel, M. A. 15
Buber, M. 123
Buytendjik, F. J. J. 113

Cady, J. W. 12, 49, 107, 126
Cartwright, A. 18, 62
Cassel, E. J. 5
Chapman, C. R. 34
Childs, G. E. 109
CIBA Foundation 71
Copp, L. A. 11, 47, 53, 104, 121
Cousins, N. 55
Crowley, D. M. 38, 121

Dally, P. 60

Daudet, A. 121
Davitz, J. 92, 99
Davitz, L. J. 92, 99
Degenaar, J. J. 113, 137
Descartes, R. 3
Dick-Read, G. 50
Diers, D. 94

Egbert, L. D. 20
Eland, J. M. 71, 74, 75
Engel, G. L. 13, 35, 37
Essex, R. 135, 136
Evely, L. 12
Everhart, D. 121

Fleck, S. 17
Frankl, V. 47, 128, 129, 131
Freud, A. 51, 72, 78, 110

Geyman, J. 32
Gibran, K. 131
Gillis, L. 17
Gomez, J. 60
Gracely, R. H. 27
Guthrie, G. J. 14

Hadlock, 61
Haslam, D. R. 71
Hayward, J. 18, 106
Hick, J. 5
Hinton, J. 39, 46, 67, 135
Hippocrates 47
Hugel, B. von 54
Hunt, J. 62
Huxley, A. 16

Illich, I. 19, 112
Ingham, J. G. 59
Ischlondsky, N. E. 47, 49

General Index

144